HILLCREST
MEDICAL CENTER
BEGINNING MEDICAL TRANSCRIPTION COURSE

SIXTH EDITION

Patricia A. Ireland, CMT, FAAMT
Medical Transcriptionist, On-Line
Instructor, Freelance Author,
Medical/Technical Editor
San Antonio, Texas

Mary Ann Novak, Ph.D.
Associate Professor, Emerita
Information Management Systems
College of Applied Sciences and Arts
Southern Illinois University
Carbondale, Illinois

THOMSON

DELMAR LEARNING™ Australia • Canada • Mexico • Singapore • Spain • United Kingdom • United States

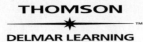

THOMSON

DELMAR LEARNING

Hillcrest Medical Center: Beginning Medical Transcription Course
Sixth Edition
by Patricia A. Ireland and Mary Ann Novak

**Vice President,
Health Care Business Unit:**
William Brottmiller

Editorial Director:
Cathy L. Esperti

Acquisitions Editor:
Maureen Rosener

Developmental Editor:
Darcy M. Scelsi

Editorial Assistant:
Elizabeth Howe

Marketing Director:
Jennifer McAvey

Marketing Channel Manager:
Lisa Stover

Technology Project Manager:
Victoria Moore

Project Editor:
David Buddle

Production Coordinator:
Kenneth McGrath

Art and Design Specialist:
Connie Lundberg-Watkins

Art and Design Coordinator:
Alexandros Vasilakos

Library of Congress Cataloging-in-Publication Data
Ireland, Patricia A., 1940–
  Hillcrest Medical Center : beginning medical transcription course / Patricia A. Ireland, Mary Ann Novak.—6th ed.
     p. cm.
  Previous ed. cataloged under: Novak, Mary A., 1944–
     Includes index.
     ISBN 1-4018-4108-2
  1. Medical transcription. I. Title: Beginning medical transcription course. II. Novak, Mary Ann, 1944– III. Novak, Mary Ann, 1944– Hillcrest Medical Center. IV. Title.
     R728.8.N68 2005
     653'.18—dc22
                                    2004045512

Notice to the Reader
Publisher does not warrant or guarantee any of the products described herein or perform any independent analysis in connection with any of the product information contained herein. Publisher does not assume, and expressly disclaims, any obligation to obtain and include information other than that provided to it by the manufacturer.

The reader is expressly warned to consider and adopt all safety precautions that might be indicated by the activities described herein and to avoid all potential hazards. By following the instructions contained herein, the reader willingly assumes all risks in connection with such instructions.

The publisher makes no representations or warranties of any kind, including but not limited to, the warranties of fitness for particular purpose or merchantability, nor are any such representations implied with respect to the material set forth herein, and the publisher takes no responsibility with respect to such material. The publisher shall not be liable for any special, consequential, or exemplary damages resulting, in whole or part, from the reader's use of, or reliance upon, this material.

Contents

Hillcrest Medical Center: Beginning Medical Transcription Course is a text-workbook created to introduce students to the interesting and challenging world of medical transcription. The contents of the text-workbook are designed to familiarize students with basic medical reports concerning Hillcrest Medical Center inpatients and Quali-Care Clinic outpatients, related medical terminology, appropriate formats for transcribing the reports, and specialized rules of grammar and punctuation peculiar to dictated medical reports. Users will apply these principles as they transcribe the medical reports that comprise the ten case studies relating to inpatients, the 25 reports relating to outpatients, and their related correspondence.

Students of the *Hillcrest Medical Center* textbook and audio-transcription exercises learn through a well-rounded course of beginning medical dictation and transcription. After the completion of this textbook, students may progress to the advanced dictation available through *Forrest General Medical Center: Advanced Medical Terminology and Transcription Course,* 3rd edition textbook and audio-transcription exercises. This advanced text goes into detailed specialty and subspecialty dictation. The *Forrest General* text is strongly recommended to round out the medical transcription students' experience and to prepare them for employment.

Prerequisites

Students should be proficient in keyboarding and have a working knowledge of transcription equipment before beginning this course. English grammar and punctuation is another important part of transcription in which the spoken word is turned into the written word. Even though a section of the text-workbook relates to understanding medical terminology, it is strongly suggested that students complete a course in medical terminology before beginning *Hillcrest Medical Center.*

Course Description

This is a beginning medical transcription course designed to provide students with a working knowledge of the transcription of medical reports. Medical reports will be transcribed from ten individual case studies, each of which concerns an inpatient with a specific medical problem. There are between four and eight reports within each case study. The case studies have been taken from hospital medical records. Students will be involved in the care of the patient from the date of admission to Hillcrest Medical

Center through the date of discharge. The medical reports include history and physical examinations, radiology reports, operative reports, pathology reports, requests for consultation, death summaries, discharge summaries, and autopsy reports. Following are the case numbers and related specialty areas.

Case 1: Reproductive System

Case 2: Musculoskeletal System

Case 3: Cardiopulmonary System

Case 4: Integumentary System

Case 5: Urinary System

Case 6: Nervous System

Case 7: Digestive System

Case 8: Endocrine System

Case 9: Lymphatic System

Case 10: Respiratory System

In addition, 25 outpatient medical reports and correspondence will be transcribed, each of which concerns a patient with a specific medical problem and who was treated by a physician at Quali-Care Clinic. The outpatient reports and correspondence have been taken from actual patient medical records. Following are the report numbers and related specialty areas.

Report 1: Gynecology Operative Report

Report 2: Pathology Report

Report 3: Cytology Report

Report 4: Oncology Consult

Report 5: Infectious Disease SOAP Note

Report 6: Pulmonology Procedure Note

Report 7: Oncology Consult

Report 8: Correspondence

Report 9: Infectious Disease Consult

Report 10: Pediatrics—Emergency Center Report

Report 11: Internal Medicine History and Physical

Report 12: Psychiatry Consult

Report 13: Radiology—Echocardiogram Report

Report 14: Radiology—Colonoscopy Procedure Note

Report 15: Radiology—CT Scan of Abdomen

Report 16: Infectious Disease HPIP Note

Report 17: Radiology—Mammogram and CT Scan of Abdomen

- *Traditional classroom setting:* These materials are designed to be effective in a traditional classroom setting. Laboratory time could be scheduled either individually or in groups. Each instructor would decide whether to be present in the lab. Estimated time to complete the case studies is 32 class hours (2 hours per week for 16 weeks) plus additional laboratory time to transcribe the medical reports (approximately 3 to 6 hours per case study). Transcription times will vary according to the length of the case study, the student's keyboarding skills, and the student's command of the English language, grammar, and punctuation. Additional lab hours should be assigned to transcribe the 25 outpatient reports and correspondence.

- *Hospital in-service education:* These materials would also be effective in a hospital in-service education department. New employees or those being cross-trained or retrained could complete the case studies plus the outpatient reports and correspondence. Those interested in a particular medical specialty could transcribe the reports related to that specialty or subspecialty area. Transcription lab time should be provided, allowing each employee to work at a comfortable pace, along with adequate feedback.

- *Online teaching:* Working equally well in a hands-on approach as in an independent-study approach, these materials are excellent when used in teaching over the internet. The same basic principles would apply with certain, obvious differences. An experienced mentor or facilitator assigned to each student would offer the proper guidance, feedback, and grading. Good communication is the key to successful teaching, whether online or otherwise. Allowing about 160 hours to complete the course, at 10 hours per week, adds up to 16 weeks.

Objectives

Upon successful completion of this course, students should be able to do the following.

1. Describe the importance of the confidential nature of medical reports. Be aware of HIPAA guidelines for the MT.

2. Describe the content and purpose of the types of inpatient medical reports used at Hillcrest Medical Center.

3. Describe the content and purpose of the 25 outpatient medical reports and correspondence used at Quali-Care Clinic.

4. Transcribe medical reports using correct report format.

5. Transcribe medical reports using correct capitalization, number, punctuation, abbreviation, symbol, and metric measurement rules.

6. Spell correctly both the English and medical terms and abbreviations presented, either by memory or by using a dictionary or reference book.

7. Define the medical terms and abbreviations presented, either by memory or by using a dictionary or reference book.

8. Define the prefixes, combining forms, and suffixes presented.

9. Identify and define the knowledge, skills, abilities, and responsibilities required of a medical transcriptionist.

10. Recognize the advantages of having current reference material and be able to use it effectively.

11. Use standard proofreader's marks to edit medical reports without changing the meaning or the dictator's style.

These objectives can be achieved by reading the material presented in the text-workbook, by transcribing the medical reports, and by completing the skill-building exercises.

Student Text-Workbook

INTRODUCTION

The introduction consists of both a welcome letter addressed to students and the confidentiality policy for Hillcrest Medical Center. The purpose of the letter is to inform students about their position as a medical transcriptionist at Hillcrest and to emphasize the importance of the medical transcriptionist's role in health care. The letter also describes Hillcrest as a specific medical facility. The "Confidentiality Policy" explains how important it is for employees at Hillcrest to understand and maintain confidentiality of patient records.

Information on the American Association for Medical Transcriptionist (AAMT), a national association representing the medical transcription profession, is also presented in this section. The AAMT Medical Transcriptionist Job Description includes a position summary for three distinct professional levels for medical transcriptionists (levels 1, 2, and 3). In addition, the nature of the work and the knowledge, skills, and abilities for each professional level are included in this section of the text. The AAMT Code of Ethics is presented with information about the AAMT national certification examination.

Also presented is information regarding the Health Insurance Portability and Accountability Act (HIPAA). This act includes standards set by the U.S. government for the security and privacy of patient medical records.

UNDERSTANDING MEDICAL RECORDS

The content and purpose of the model inpatient medical report forms used at Hillcrest Medical Center are discussed in this section.

TRANSCRIPTION RULES FOR HILLCREST

Rules pertaining to capitalization, numbers, punctuation, abbreviations, and symbols used to create medical reports at both Hillcrest Medical Center and Quali-Care Clinic are discussed.

CASE STUDIES

Students will be required to complete ten case studies. Each case study consists of the following.

1. A scenario including the inpatient's name and address, a summary of the inpatient's medical problem, the various specialists involved in the inpatient's care, and a list of specific reports involved.
2. A glossary of medical terms used in each case study that includes definitions and phonetic pronunciations.
3. Pertinent illustrations.

OUTPATIENT REPORTS

Students will also be required to complete 25 outpatient reports and correspondence. Information about each outpatient includes the following.

1. The patient's name with a brief description of the patient's illness
2. A glossary of medical terms used in each outpatient report and/or letter that includes definitions and pronunciations
3. Pertinent illustrations

AUDIO TRANSCRIPTION EXERCISES

Transcription exercises are available in three formats: cassette, audio CD, and MP3 audio files downloaded from www.delmarlearning.com. The reports related to each inpatient case are to be transcribed by the students. The terms listed in each glossary are dictated, followed by the medical report dictation. Cases 1 through 5 contain timed dictation at 80 and 90 words per minute; cases 6 through 10 contain office-style dictation. Different regional accents and background noises that duplicate real-life situations are used in the recorded dictation. The ten transcription tests are dictated using the same speed and style as their corresponding case exercises.

The reports related to each outpatient are also to be transcribed by the students. The terms listed in each glossary are dictated, followed by the medical report dictation. Reports 1 through 10 contain timed dictation at 80 and 90 words per minute; reports 11 through 25 contain office-style dictation. Different regional accents and background noises that duplicate real-life situations are used in the recorded dictation. The ten transcription tests are dictated using the same speed and style as the 25 outpatient medical reports; i.e., transcription test 1 is dictated at 80 words per minute, transcription test 2 is dictated at 90 words per minute, and transcription tests 3 through 10 contain office-style dictation.

SKILL-BUILDING EXERCISES

Additional exercises are included in the Appendix to strengthen students' skills in medical transcription. These include proofreading exercises and crossword puzzles.

APPENDIX

The following helpful information is included in the Appendix.

Proofreader's Marks

Challenging Medical Words, Phrases, Prefixes

Sample Patient History Form

The Lund Browder Chart

Laboratory Test Information

Sample Forms for Ordering Laboratory Tests, Radiology Tests and Consults, Medical Supplies

Building a Reference Library

Transcription Websites

"A Healthcare Controlled Vocabulary" by Dr. Neil Davis

How to Use the Student Activities CD-ROM

INDEX

The words, phrases, and abbreviations listed in each glossary are presented in alphabetic order in the index, along with the prefixes, combining forms, and suffixes. The page numbers identify their first location in the text-workbook.

NOTE: The terms presented *within* the Hillcrest Medical Center glossaries and *within* the Quali-Care Clinic glossaries are not duplicated. However, Hillcrest Medical Center and Quali-Care Clinic are separate entities; therefore, duplicate terms will exist between the Hillcrest Medical Center and Quali-Care Clinic glossaries.

Instructor's Manual

A comprehensive Instructor's Manual is available that discusses the design of the course, suggestions for teaching the course, evaluation procedures, and production standards. Transcripts for the ten inpatient case studies and the 25 outpatient medical reports and correspondence are provided in the manual, as well as a test bank that includes the following.

1. Ten written quizzes plus the answer keys, which correlate with the ten inpatient case studies.

2. The answer keys to ten transcription tests relating to inpatient case studies, which are recorded on the audio transcription exercises.

3. The answer keys to ten transcription tests relating to outpatients, which are recorded on the audio transcription exercises.

4. Answer keys to the proofreading exercises and crossword puzzles.

An Instructor's Resource CD-ROM containing Microsoft Word files of every report in the *Instructor's Manual* is included in the back of the manual. The CD-ROM allows instructors to make electronic comparisons of the students' transcription to the original, correct reports. This allows instructors to easily recognize student errors. For help using the comparison feature, please refer to the help menus in Microsoft Word.

A Certificate of Completion, to be given to the student on successful completion of *Hillcrest Medical Center,* is also included in the manual.

ACKNOWLEDGMENTS

This text-workbook is the result of the cooperation and input of many individuals. The authors would like to express their appreciation for authentic medical reports submitted for adaptation and inclusion in this text-workbook. Additionally, the authors want to thank the reviewers for their contributions and suggestions. Their feedback enabled us to develop a text-workbook to better serve your needs.

Tricia Berry, OTR/L
Medical Program Coordinator
Hamilton College
Des Moines, IA

Barbara A. Blank, CMT
The Toledo Hospital
Toledo, OH

Cindi Brassington, MS, CMA
Quinebaug Valley Community College
Danielson, CT

John H. Dirckx, MD
Dayton, OH

Gisele Dubson, BA, CMT
Front Range Community College
Mercury Medical Communications
Boulder, CO

Karen Griffin
Forsyth Technical Community College
Winston Salem, NC

Cheryl Hammel, RN, CMT
Southern Illinois Healthcare

Joyce Minton, BS, CMA, RMA
Wilkes Community College
Wilkesboro, NC

Dorothy Reinhart, BS
Medical Careers Institute
Newport News, VA

Carrie Stein, CMT
San Antonio, TX
(With her expertise, Ms. Stein advised us time and again and has been a source of inspiration.)

Darlene M. Walker, CEO
Report Works, A Medical Transcription Service
Sylmar, CA

Reviewers of past editions:

Linda Andrews
Director
The Andrews School
Oklahoma City, OK

Shirley S. Gordon
Instructor
Ascension College
Gonzales, LA

Brenda Potter
Medical Secretary Instructor
Moorhead Northwest Technical Institute
Fargo, ND

Esther Storvold
Selkirk College
Trail, BC

Barbara Thomas
Salisbury Business College
Salisbury, NC

Mary Walker
Southwestern Technical College
Jackson, MN

About the Authors

Patricia A. Ireland, CMT, FAAMT, has been in medical transcription since 1968 as both a practitioner and instructor. She lives in San Antonio, Texas, working as a medical transcriptionist, a freelance medical and technical editor, and an instructor for an online medical terminology and medical transcription teaching program.

Mary Ann Novak, PhD, has been teaching office professionals for 23 years and is Associate Professor Emerita in the Department of Information Management Services, College of Applied Sciences and Arts, Southern Illinois University, Carbondale, Illinois.

How to Use the Student Activities CD-ROM to Accompany
Hillcrest Medical Center: Beginning Medical Transcription Course, Sixth Edition

Use this program as your own private tutor to help you learn the material in your *Hillcrest Medical Center: Beginning Medical Transcription Course*, Sixth Edition, text-workbook.

Menus

You can access any of the menus from wherever you are in the program. The menus include Quizzes, Scores, Activities, and Templates.

Quizzes

Quizzes include multiple-choice, true-false, and word-building questions. You can take the quizzes in both Practice Mode and Quiz Mode. Use Practice Mode to improve your mastery of the material. You have multiple tries to get the answers correct and are assisted by hints on wrong answers. Use Quiz Mode when you are ready to test yourself and keep a record of your scores. In Quiz Mode, you have one try to get the answers right and you cannot change your answers once you have submitted them.

Scores

You can view your last scores for each quiz and print your results to hand in to your instructor.

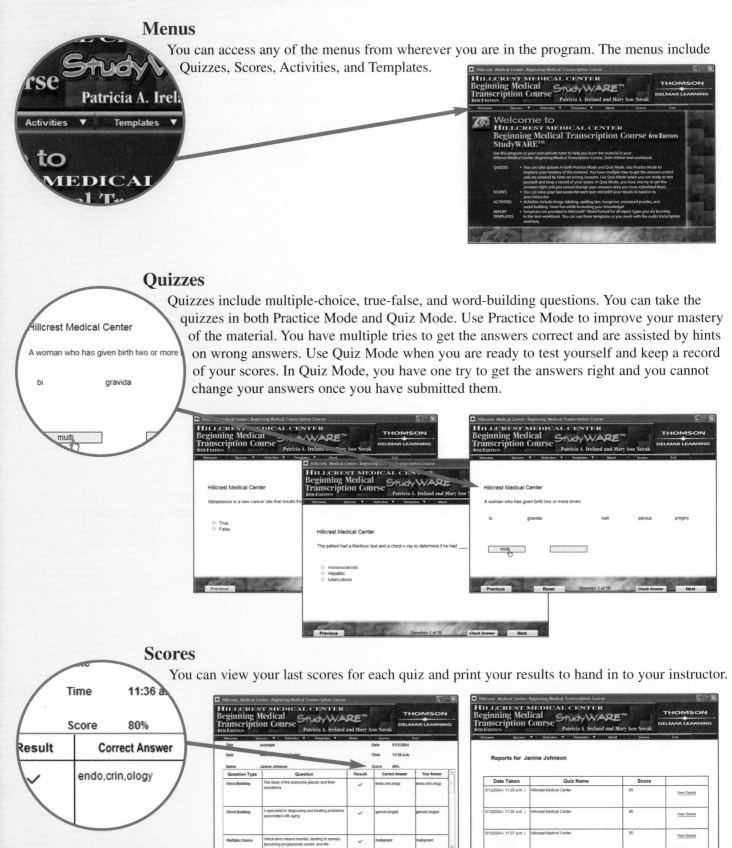

Activities

Activities include image labeling, spelling bee, hangman, and crossword puzzles. Have fun while increasing your knowledge!

Report Templates

Templates are provided in Microsoft Word format for all report types you are learning in the text-workbook. You can use these templates as you work with the audio transcription exercises.

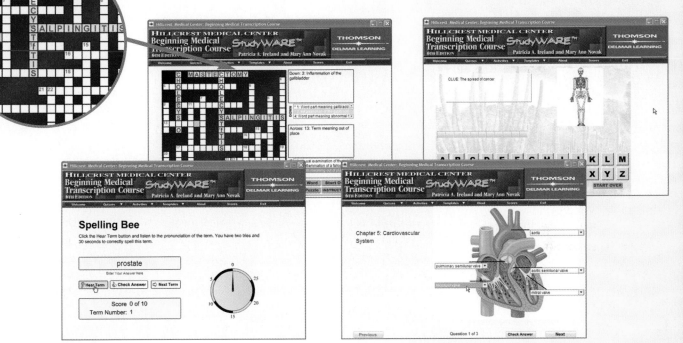

SECTION 1
Introduction

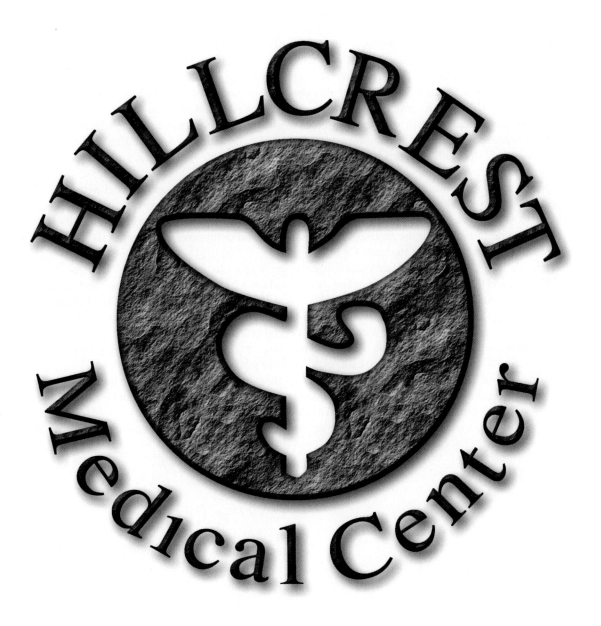

You are now employed as a medical transcriptionist (MT) in the information management department at Hillcrest Medical Center, transcribing reports for patients admitted to Hillcrest Medical Center and transcribing outpatient reports for patients treated at Quali-Care Clinic. MTs are a vital part of the healthcare team because physicians and allied health professionals rely on medical records, legal documents subject to subpoena, to maintain and document proper patient care. Because of the confidential nature of these medical records, you will be asked to read the "Confidentiality Policy" on page 3 and sign the "Confidentiality Statement" before beginning your duties at Hillcrest.

During your employment at Hillcrest, you will be transcribing medical reports from ten individual case studies, each relating to an inpatient with a specific medical problem. The case studies have been taken from actual hospital medical records, and you will be involved in the care of each patient from the date of admission to Hillcrest through the date of discharge. The types of medical reports you will be transcribing include history and physical examinations, radiology reports, operative reports, pathology reports, requests for consultation, discharge summaries, death summaries, and autopsy reports.

Presented on the first page of each case study is a brief scenario including the patient's name and address, a summary of the patient's medical problem, the various specialists involved in the patient's care, and a list of the specific reports involved. In addition, a glossary of medical terms is provided for each case study. Each glossary includes phonetic pronunciations with definitions for the medical terms, phrases, and abbreviations used in each case study.

The MTs who are employed by Hillcrest will also transcribe dictated tapes for the health care providers who maintain offices at Quali-Care Clinic. This service is provided as a courtesy to the staff of Quali-Care Clinic, a freestanding medical office facility on the grounds of Hillcrest Medical Center. With the changes in insurance, the advent of health management organizations, preferred provider organizations, and managed care, the Hillcrest Medical Center Board of Directors voted to have Quali-Care Clinic built to treat a burgeoning number of outpatients—those who have no need for either inpatient care or emergency room care.

The performance evaluations in this text-workbook will consist of transcription tests and written quizzes. Therefore, it is important to learn the information presented in each case study and medical report, including appropriate report format and transcription rules observed by the Hillcrest information management department. Before transcribing the medical reports, become familiar with the spellings, pronunciations, and definitions of the terms and abbreviations presented in the glossaries. Words are tools of the trade for MTs.

Hillcrest Medical Center is a 400-bed general community hospital located in Miami, Florida. All patient services, the emergency room, and the surgery suite are found on the first and second floors. On the third floor are beds for 60 inpatients—20 in the pediatric unit, 20 in the coronary care unit (CCU), and 20 in the intensive care unit (ICU). Pediatric patients are usually those 14 years of age or younger. CCU is for patients—medical or surgical—who are seriously ill with heart disease; an ICU patient is either gravely ill or has had surgery on a weekend or a holiday. Otherwise, the postoperative patients are sent to the fourth floor where there are 100 beds for surgical patients. The fifth floor has 100 beds used for medical patients, and the sixth floor has 100 beds used for geriatric patients or for those who need long-term care.

From time to time Hillcrest accepts patients transferred from Forrest General Hospital, the county hospital and teaching facility for the local medical school. Hillcrest sometimes sends patients to Forrest General for specific evaluations, consultations, or certain sophisticated procedures not available at Hillcrest.

We look forward to a pleasant working relationship, and we hope your employment as an MT at Hillcrest Medical Center proves to be a rewarding experience.

Sincerely,

Allison Poole

Allison Poole, CMT, RHIA
Director, Information Management Department

Confidentiality Policy

The primary purpose of the medical record is to document the course of a patient's illness and treatment during all periods of the patient's care. The medical record is extremely important as a permanent account of the patient care provided. It serves as a means of communication between physicians and other health care professionals. As such, it is also a tool for planning and evaluating patient care.

For the medical record to be a useful instrument in patient care, it must contain accurate, detailed, personal information relating to each patient's medical, surgical, psychiatric, social, and family history.

Patients have the *right* to expect their medical records to be treated as *confidential,* and Hillcrest Medical Center personnel have an *obligation* to safeguard patients' medical records against unauthorized disclosure.

As an employee of Hillcrest Medical Center, you have a responsibility to ensure that each patient's right to privacy is safeguarded. You will have direct access to information contained in medical records. Information learned during the course of your work *must* be held in strictest confidence.

To ensure the confidentiality of patient information, employees of Hillcrest Medical Center must sign a statement acknowledging this confidentiality policy and must attend an orientation session regarding HIPAA. Violations of this policy will result in immediate disciplinary action.

CONFIDENTIALITY STATEMENT

I, _____, an employee of Hillcrest Medical Center, have read and reviewed the Confidentiality Policy with my supervisor. I understand the importance of each employee complying with this policy. I further understand that if I intentionally violate this policy by any unauthorized release of a patient's medical information, this violation could constitute grounds for my immediate dismissal.

_____	_____
Date	Signature of Employee
_____	_____
Date	Witness

Legal Issues

In creating these medical reports, which are legal documents, what do you do if dictation is unintelligible or a section is blank? Students and experienced MTs both encounter dictation that cannot be understood, and a directive should be in place in each MT's office or workplace in this event. Some suggestions follow.

1. If you encounter a word or phrase that is unfamiliar, look it up in your reference material.

This would include dictionaries, word books, drug books, and other lists of medical words/phrases. (See Reference Material, page 39).

2. If you are unsuccessful in locating the word or phrase in the reference material, have your supervisor or a coworker listen to the difficult section of dictation. One of them may be able to interpret the word or phrase.

3. If these two options are unsuccessful, the report should be flagged for the originator's attention. An underlined blank (_____) should *always* be left when dictation is left out of a report. This lets anyone who comes in contact with the report know that there is a question about the dictation—words to be filled in—and the originator of the report is the one to fill in the word(s).

A telephone call to the doctor's office could possibly yield results; however, this is not always feasible. As you work in the field of medical transcription, you will learn different tricks of the trade that can be used. As beginners, however, you must follow your supervisor's lead. The ideal report, of course, has no blanks; however, this situation is often out of the MT's control. Even so, you should *not* make up words to avoid leaving a blank. Even experienced MTs leave blanks from time to time.

The physician who originates the report and whose signature is on it is the party legally responsible for the contents thereof. This means that each report should be carefully read by the originator, corrected in the computer, reprinted, then signed as corrected. Unfortunately, this is another situation that is not within the MT's control. The originator may make handwritten corrections on the report that never get back to the transcriptionist and, therefore, never get entered into the computer. Also, many reports are signed without being read at all. This includes electronic signatures, examples of which are in this text. Some institutions employ an electronic signature that includes the statement, "Signed but not read." So, even though the originator is legally responsible, more and more MTs are buying liability (sometimes called errors and omissions) insurance to cover themselves in case of a lawsuit. (The cost of this insurance would be a valid business tax deduction.)

Health Insurance Portability and Accountability Act (HIPAA)

Security and privacy have a continual role in medicine. The health care arena has likewise been aware of the patient's right to protect his or her medical information. Until the information age, patients assumed that medical personnel would be vigilant about keeping information secure and confidential. With one click of a button, however, the internet now allows confidential information to travel worldwide. With that and a mobile America, the U.S. government determined that health care portability and confidentiality should be mandated and regulated.

Whether working as a medical transcriptionist in the hospital setting, clinic, or physician's office, as an employee or independent contractor, HIPAA regulations will definitely impact the way you do your job. As an MT, you are entrusted with patient information, even if just for a short time, and your job is to treat that information as you would want your own personal medical information treated.

Be aware of patients' rights with regard to confidentiality of medical information, stay abreast of federal and state regulations and the changes that may take place, and respect the confidence that has been placed in your competence as a health care professional.

For further information, AAMT offers a brochure on the HIPAA regulations at www.aamt.org.

Objectives

At Hillcrest Medical Center, students learn how to transcribe medical reports. During the transcription process, students will increase their medical vocabulary, use an appropriate format for transcribing the reports, and apply specialized rules of grammar and punctuation peculiar to dictated medical reports. Upon successful completion of this course, students should be able to do the following.

1. Describe the importance of the confidential nature of medical records.
2. Describe the content and purpose of the medical inpatient reports used at Hillcrest Medical Center.
3. Describe the content and purpose of the outpatient medical reports and correspondence used at Quali-Care Clinic.
4. Transcribe medical reports using correct report format.
5. Transcribe medical reports using correct capitalization, number, punctuation, abbreviation, symbol, and metric measurement rules.
6. Spell correctly both the English and medical terms and abbreviations presented, either by memory or by using a dictionary/reference book.
7. Define the medical terms and abbreviations presented, either by memory or by using a dictionary/reference book.
8. Define the prefixes, combining forms, and suffixes presented.
9. Identify and define the knowledge, skills, abilities, and responsibilities required of an MT.
10. Recognize the advantages of having current reference material and be able to use it effectively.

11. Use standard proofreader's marks to edit medical reports without changing the meaning or the originator's style.

These objectives can be achieved by reading the material presented in the text-workbook, by transcribing the medical reports, and by completing the proofreading exercises.

Length of Course

Students will be required to complete the ten inpatient case studies listed below. The time estimated to complete the case studies is 32 class hours (2 days per week for 16 weeks), plus additional laboratory time to transcribe the medical reports (approximately 3 to 6 hours per case study). Transcription time will vary depending on the length of the case study, the student's keyboarding skills, and the student's command of English language usage, punctuation, and transcription guidelines.

Case 1:   Reproductive System
Case 2:   Musculoskeletal System
Case 3:   Cardiopulmonary System
Case 4:   Integumentary System
Case 5:   Urinary System
Case 6:   Nervous System
Case 7:   Digestive System
Case 8:   Endocrine System
Case 9:   Lymphatic System
Case 10:   Respiratory System

Additional laboratory time should be allotted to the students to transcribe the 25 outpatient medical reports and correspondence, each of which concerns a patient with a specific medical problem treated by a physician at Quali-Care Clinic. The outpatient reports and correspondence have been taken from actual patient medical records. Following are the report numbers and related specialty areas.

Report 1:   Gynecology Operative Report
Report 2:   Pathology Report
Report 3:   Cytology Report
Report 4:   Oncology Consult
Report 5:   Infectious Disease SOAP Note
Report 6:   Pulmonology Procedure Note
Report 7:   Oncology Consult
Report 8:   Correspondence
Report 9:   Infectious Disease Consult
Report 10: Pediatrics—Emergency Center Report
Report 11: Internal Medicine History and Physical
Report 12: Psychiatry Consult
Report 13: Radiology—Echocardiogram Report

CERTIFICATION

The word *certification* is used in different ways. A certificate of completion is offered after almost any course that you may take. This certifies that you have completed the required course work, and it may be beneficial to have for your résumé or personnel file. It does not mean, however, that you are a certified medical transcriptionist (CMT).

Certification by your professional association, which for MTs is the American Association for Medical Transcription currently in Modesto, California, is much different. You earn status as a CMT by passing both the written and practical examinations offered by AAMT. Earning 30 continuing education credits every three years, which are reported to AAMT on specialized forms, retains certification.

Certification is not required for AAMT membership or to work in the field of medical transcription. It is, however, a mark of quality and professionalism that indicates a dedication to continuing education.

In addition to certification, a medical transcriptionist can become recognized as a fellow of AAMT. To earn fellow status, the applicant must earn at least 50 fellowship points in the five years immediately preceding the application. Points may be earned in eight different categories, demonstrating a balance between practice duties, professional experience, leadership, and community involvement.

Transcribing Medical Reports

A medical record objectively records the patient's clinical course from evaluation through treatment. A clear, accurate medical record confirms what was done and not done.

Review the following information prior to transcribing the medical reports presented in this text-workbook.

1. Become familiar with the content and format of the Hillcrest Medical Center inpatient model report forms. Also become familiar with the content and format of the Quali-Care Clinic outpatient model report forms. The structure of outpatient and inpatient medical reports will vary among health care facilities.

2. Become familiar with the prefixes, combining forms, and suffixes that begin on page 53.

3. Learn the spelling and definition of the medical terms, phrases, and abbreviations presented in the glossary preceding each inpatient case study and each outpatient medical report or letter. The glossaries in the case studies and medical reports are cumulative. Medical terms and abbreviations can have more than one meaning and more than one pronunciation; the definitions presented here pertain to the Hillcrest case studies and the Quali-Care medical reports and correspondence.

4. The medical terms, phrases, and abbreviations appearing in the glossaries are dictated on the audio transcription exercises that accompany the text-workbook. Listen to the pronunciation of these terms prior to transcribing each case study. Take time to become familiar with the sound of each word.

5. The pronunciation of most medical terms is indicated by a phonetic respelling that appears in parentheses immediately following each term in the glossary.

6. Prior to transcribing, review the rules of capitalization, numbers, punctuation, abbreviations, and symbols on pages 41–45. These rules are not all inclusive, and it is recommended that you use one of the standard grammar reference books.

7. Maintain at least 1-inch side margins and 1-inch top and bottom margins on each transcribed page.

8. If an inpatient medical report consists of more than one page, each succeeding page should have a heading at the left margin to include the name of the report. (See model reports for an example of a second-page heading.) If an outpatient medical report consists of more than one page, each succeeding page should have a heading that includes patient name, date seen, and page number. Second- and third-page headings may vary among health care facilities.

9. At the end of each report, key a signature line for the physician who dictated the report. Transcriptionist sign-off information consists of the reference initials of both the originator and transcriptionist, the date the report was dictated (D), and the date transcribed (T). This is keyed at the left margin two spaces below the signature line. (See model reports for an example of a signature line and transcriptionist sign-off information.)

10. In the case of pathology reports, the gross description is usually done on the day of scheduled surgery. The microscopic description and diagnosis are done after the tissue removed at surgery has been properly processed (at least 24 hours later). Therefore, the reference initials and dates dictated and transcribed are recorded after the gross description and again after the microscopic description and diagnosis unless it is a "gross only" report. The physician and MT for the two descriptions may be the same or they may be different. Whether the same or different physicians dictate the gross description and the microscopic description, two sets of reference initials and dates are required with one signature line at the end of the report. (See pathology model report.)

Evaluations

Upon completion of each inpatient case study, you are required to take a written quiz that consists of the terms and their definitions as presented in each glossary. Each quiz is worth 20 points.

Ten transcription tests that relate to inpatients at Hillcrest and ten transcription tests that relate to outpatients at Quali-Care are included on the audio transcription exercises. Your instructor will decide when to administer the transcription tests; however, it is advisable to have transcribed and received feedback on at least the first two inpatient case studies and the first five outpatient reports before being assigned a transcription test.

Skill-Building Exercises

The skill-building exercises have been provided to increase your proficiency in both medical terminology and medical transcription.

CROSSWORD PUZZLES

In keeping with the idea of being "word people," or those who find pleasure in working with and playing with words, Hillcrest offers six crossword puzzles to reinforce knowledge of terms presented in "Understanding Medical Terminology" in Section 3 (see pages 53–61) as well as the terms presented in the ten inpatient case glossaries.

The crossword puzzles are offered as an alternate group activity. They are not intended to be used as testing material or as homework assignments, but as activities to be completed from memory.

PROOFREADING EXERCISES

"Detail oriented" is a phrase that describes an MT. "Focal" and "word person" are others. In creating and editing medical records, students should strive to become detail-oriented, focal workers.

The MT makes several key decisions while at work: choosing the correct medical word by meaning and context, the correct spelling for both medical terms and English words, the correct format according to institution or client, punctuation, grammar, spacing, styling of numbers and symbols, *plus* editing, i.e., making additions and deletions without changing either the meaning or the originator's style.

To help beginning MT students become focal, detail-oriented professionals, Hillcrest offers a set of proofreading exercises. Errors incorporated into these exercises include examples of all the key decisions to be made by an MT. The standard proofreader's marks are printed on page 190. Using them will help MT students learn the fundamentals of proofreading and marking changes on an edited medical report. (*Note:* Not all the errors included would be caught by spellcheck. No student or practitioner should depend solely on spellcheck. Nothing takes the place of carefully proofreading your work.)

Appendix

The following information is included in the Appendix.

1. Proofreader's marks
2. Challenging medical words, phrases, prefixes
3. Sample patient history form
4. Lund Browder chart
5. Laboratory test information
6. Sample forms for ordering lab tests, radiology tests, and consults
7. Building a reference library
8. Transcription websites
9. "A Healthcare Controlled Vocabulary" by Dr. Neil Davis

CHALLENGING MEDICAL WORDS, PHRASES, AND PREFIXES

This list, developed over years of transcribing and teaching medical transcription students, represents difficult words that trouble many health care workers and MTs. It is helpful to remove the list and keep at your workstation for quick referral, adding to the list as necessary.

LUND BROWDER BURN CHART

The Lund Browder burn chart is used in hospitals and burn centers especially for pediatric burn patients. This standard chart shows the anterior and posterior aspects of the human body divided into segments. It is used to estimate the percentage of burned body tissue area. One of these charts is used on admission and at each debridement, which is a surgical procedure wherein both foreign material and contaminated tissue are removed, exposing healthy tissue. The Lund Browder chart is also used to show areas used as donor sites plus those areas covered with skin grafts and other types of grafts or dressings. This provides an ongoing picture of the progress in covering burn wounds. Published many years ago, this chart is widely used to help provide proper care for burn patients.

A "HEALTHCARE CONTROLLED VOCABULARY"

The safety principles regarding language used by health care professionals, as described in the article, "A Healthcare Controlled Vocabulary," by Dr. Neil Davis, are important for all MTs to understand. Dr. Davis is a pioneer in promoting these principles.

The American Association for Medical Transcription (AAMT), which represents the medical transcription profession, defines an MT as a medical language specialist who interprets and transcribes dictation by physicians and other health care professionals regarding patient assessment, workup, therapeutic procedures, clinical course, diagnosis, prognosis, etc., to document patient care and facilitate delivery of health care services.

AAMT has created the Medical Transcriptionist Job Descriptions analysis, based on a study conducted by the Hay Management Consultants, which defines three distinct professional levels for medical transcriptionists.

MEDICAL TRANSCRIPTIONIST JOB DESCRIPTIONS
Results of a Benchmarking Analysis of MT Professional Levels

PROFESSIONAL LEVELS

In an independent benchmarking study of the medical transcription profession by the Hay Management Consultants (Hay Group), three distinct professional levels for medical transcriptionists were identified and described in the following table. The Hay Group is a worldwide human resources consulting firm with extensive expertise in work analysis and job measurement.

COMPENSATION

Subsequent to this benchmark study of the job content levels of MTs, the Hay Group conducted a compensation survey, analyzing pay as it relates to these levels. (Hay's survey methodology complied with federal antitrust regulations regarding health care compensation surveys.) The results include information on transcription pay at the corporate level (health care organizations and MT businesses) and compensation for independent contractors. The data are further presented by geographic region, size of business, types of pay programs (pay for time worked and pay for production), and reward programs (benefits, etc.). The Hay report, "Compensation for Medical Transcriptionists," is contained in a 30-page booklet, available from AAMT.

American Association for Medical Transcription Code of Ethics Adopted July 10, 1995

PART I: ASSOCIATION MEMBERSHIP

Preamble

Be aware that it is by our standards of conduct and professionalism that the American Association for Medical Transcription (AAMT) is evaluated. As members of AAMT we should recognize and observe the goals and objectives of the organization and the limitations and confinements imposed by its bylaws, policies, and procedures.

Scope of Member Conduct

AAMT members (in individual categories of membership) will

1. Place the goals and purposes of the Association above personal gain and work for the good of the profession.
2. Discharge honorably and to the best of their ability the responsibility of any elected or appointed Association position.
3. Preserve the confidential nature of professional judgments and determinations made confidentially by the official bodies of the Association.
4. Represent truthfully and accurately (a) one's membership in the association, (b) one's roles and functions in the association, and (c) any positions and decisions of the association.

PART II: PROFESSIONAL STANDARDS

Preamble

AAMT members are aware that it is by our standards of conduct and professionalism that the entire profession of medical transcription is evaluated. We should conduct ourselves in the practice of our profession so as to bring dignity and honor to ourselves and to the profession of medical transcription as medical language specialists. Therefore, the following standards are considered essential in the workplace.

1. A medical transcriptionist undertakes work only if she/he is competent to perform it.

2. A medical transcriptionist exhibits honesty and integrity in his/her professional work and activities.

3. A medical transcriptionist is reasonably familiar with and complies with principles of accuracy, authenticity, privacy, confidentiality, and security concerning patient care information.

4. A medical transcriptionist engages in professional reading and continuing education sufficient to stay abreast of important professional information.

5. A medical transcriptionist does not misrepresent or falsify information concerning medical records, his/her fees, work or professional experience, credentials, or affiliations.

6. A medical transcriptionist complies with applicable law and professional standards governing his/her work.

7. A medical transcriptionist does not assist others to violate ethical principles or professional standards of the medical transcription field.

8. If a medical transcriptionist learns of a significant unethical practice by another medical transcriptionist, she/he takes reasonable steps to resolve the matter.

9. A medical transcriptionist who agrees to serve in an official capacity in a professional association exhibits honesty and integrity in discharging his/her responsibilities.

10. AAMT members who are not medical transcriptionists should abide by the above principles where applicable.[1]

[1]*Copyright 1995. Reprinted with permission of American Association for Medical Transcription, Modesto, CA.*

MEDICAL TRANSCRIPTIONIST JOB DESCRIPTION		
	Professional Level 1	**Professional Level 2**	**Professional Level 3**
Position Summary	Medical language specialist who transcribes dictation by physicians and other health care providers to document patient care. The incumbent will likely need assistance to interpret dictation that is unclear or inconsistent, or make use of professional reference materials.	Medical language specialist who transcribes and interprets dictation by physicians and other health care providers to document patient care. The position is also routinely involved in research of questions and in the education of others involved with patient care documentation.	Medical language specialist whose expert depth and breadth of professional experience enables him or her to serve as a medical language resource to originators, coworkers, other health care providers, and/or students on a regular basis.
Nature of Work	An incumbent in this position is given assignments that are matched to his or her developing skill level, with the intention of increasing the depth and/or breadth of exposure. OR The nature of the work performed (type of report or correspondence, medical specialty, originator) is repetitive or patterned, not requiring extensive depth and/or breadth of experience.	An incumbent in this position is given assignments that require a seasoned depth of knowledge in a medical specialty (or specialties). OR The incumbent is regularly given assignments that vary in report or correspondence type, originator, and specialty. Incumbents at this level are able to resolve nonroutine problems independently, or to assist in resolving complex or highly unusual problems.	An incumbent in this position routinely researches and resolves complex questions related to health information or related documentation. AND/OR The incumbent is involved in the formal teaching of those entering the profession or continuing their education in the profession. AND/OR The incumbent regularly uses extensive experience to interpret dictation that others are unable to clarify. Actual transcription of dictation is performed only occasionally, as efforts are usually focused in other categories of work.

(Continued)

	Professional Level 1	Professional Level 2	Professional Level 3
Knowledge, Skills, and Abilities	1. Basic knowledge of medical terminology, anatomy and physiology, disease processes, signs and symptoms, medications, and laboratory values. Knowledge of specialty (or specialties) as appropriate.	1. Seasoned knowledge of medical terminology, anatomy and physiology, disease processes, signs and symptoms, medications, and laboratory values. In-depth or broad knowledge of a specialty (or specialties) as appropriate.	1. Recognized as possessing expert knowledge of medical terminology, anatomy and physiology, disease processes, signs and symptoms, medications, and laboratory values related to a specialty or specialties.
	2. Knowledge of medical transcription guidelines and practices.	2. Knowledge of medical transcription guidelines and practices.	2. In-depth knowledge of medical transcription guidelines and practices.
	3. Proven skills in English usage, grammar, punctuation, style, and editing.	3. Excellent skills in English usage, grammar, punctuation, and style.	3. Excellent skills in English usage, grammar, punctuation, and style.
	4. Ability to use designated professional reference materials.	4. Ability to use an extensive array of professional reference materials.	4. Ability to use a vast array of professional reference materials, often in innovative ways.
	5. Ability to operate word processing equipment, dictation and transcription equipment, and other equipment as specified.	5. Ability to operate word processing equipment, dictation and transcription equipment, and other equipment as specified, and to troubleshoot as necessary.	5. Ability to educate others (one on one or group).
	6. Ability to work under pressure with time constraints.	6. Ability to work independently with minimal or no supervision.	6. Excellent written and oral communication skills.
	7. Ability to concentrate.	7. Ability to work under pressure with time constraints.	7. Ability to operate word processing equipment, dictation and transcription equipment, and other equipment as specified, and to troubleshoot as necessary.
	8. Excellent listening skills.	8. Ability to concentrate.	8. Proven business skills (scheduling work, purchasing, client relations, billing).
	9. Excellent eye, hand, and auditory coordination.	9. Excellent listening skills.	9. Ability to understand and apply relevant legal concepts (e.g., confidentiality).
	10. Ability to understand and apply relevant legal concepts (e.g., confidentiality).	10. Excellent eye, hand, and auditory coordination.	10. Certified medical transcriptionist (CMT) status preferred.
		11. Proven business skills (scheduling work, purchasing, client relations, billing).	
		12. Ability to understand and apply relevant legal concepts (e.g., confidentiality).	
		13. Certified medical transcriptionist (CMT) status preferred.	

Employment and Certification Possibilities

Due to the variety of skills that MTs (medical language specialists) possess, they are employable in a variety of health care settings including doctors' offices, public and private hospitals, teaching hospitals, psychiatric hospitals, radiology departments, clinics, medical transcription services, pathology laboratories, insurance companies, medical libraries, government medical facilities, publishing companies, research facilities, and in the legal profession.

Experienced MTs may become teachers working in adult education to train future MTs. They may become reviewers, authors, or editors working through the publishing process to provide new and improved medical publications including course material and reference books.

Expert MTs who want to increase their professional responsibilities beyond medical transcription may become supervisors, managers, or owners of private transcription services.

After gaining experience as an MT, preferably in a hospital medical transcription or information management department setting, one may apply to sit for the national medical transcription certification examination sponsored by AAMT. A person who successfully completes the two-part examination earns the status of certified medical transcriptionist (CMT), which is a mark of distinction in the field of medical transcription. A CMT is recognized as a dedicated, professional MT who participates in an ongoing program of continuing medical education approved by AAMT. CMTs are required to accrue 30 continuing education credit hours during a 3-year cycle to retain the CMT status.

For additional information about the medical transcription profession and the national certification examination, write the American Association for Medical Transcription, 100 Sycamore Avenue, Modesto CA 95354-0550; visit the AAMT website at www.aamt.org or contact AAMT via their e-mail address at aamt@aamt.org.

Every time a patient enters Hillcrest Medical Center or Quali-Care Clinic—through the hospital admissions department, the hospital emergency room, for day surgery, or for outpatient treatment—a detailed record of the patient's care is created. Medical records are created by physicians and other health care providers dictating the results of their findings on patients they see, test, and examine. They originate patient reports that may be dictated in patient care areas; in pathology, radiology, other departments of the hospital; in the clinic; or even offsite. The hospital medical records are the property of Hillcrest Medical Center and are kept according to the regulations of the Joint Commission on Accreditation of Healthcare Organizations (JCAHO). Patients can get copies of their medical records; however, the information contained therein is confidential. No one has a right to obtain patient files without written permission (called an authorization or a release) from the patient.

Certain circumstances require legal disclosure of confidential information to state departments of health or social services, such as the following.

1. Birth and death
2. Blindness
3. Child abuse
4. Industrial poisoning
5. Vaccinations
6. Sexually transmitted and communicable diseases
7. Injuries resulting from criminal violence
8. Requests for plastic surgery without apparent reason (e.g., changing fingerprints or something that might indicate that the patient is a fugitive from justice)

Although laws vary from state to state relative to the length of time hospital medical records should be kept, both Hillcrest and Quali-Care Clinic chose to have each patient record microfilmed and retained for 25 years after the closure of the patient file. Because Hillcrest subscribes to voluntary accreditation by JCAHO, which means the hospital submits to inspections of each department by this private, not-for-profit agency every three years and follows its guidelines, the information management department is bound by JCAHO regulations in many of their departmental and record-keeping decisions.

The following eight basic medical reports are used at Hillcrest Medical Center.

1. History and Physical Examination Reports
2. Radiology Reports
3. Operative Reports
4. Pathology Reports
5. Requests for Consultation
6. Discharge Summaries
7. Death Summaries
8. Autopsy Reports

Examples of these documents are presented in "Model Report Forms," Section 2, which begins on page 15. A brief explanation of each of these report forms follows. Additional tips for formatting your reports can be found in "Using the Student Activities CD-ROM," Section 3. The model report forms illustrate some of these guidelines.

History and Physical Examination (H&P)

When a patient is admitted to the hospital for evaluation and treatment, the admitting/attending physician prepares a medical history detailing the specific complaint/illness that prompted admission to the hospital. Information about the patient's past medical history, surgery, allergies, and family and social histories, as well as psychiatric information, may be included in this report. A review of the systems of the body (a survey of possible symptoms or historical facts relating to the patient's organs) may also be included. The content of the patient's history will vary depending on the chief complaint of the patient, on the physician's specialty, and on the physician's personal style; however, the history consists largely of subjective findings. The report of the physical examination includes vital signs and other objective findings by the physician.

The H&P is a priority item in the patient's hospital course because it is the summary of the information known at the time of admission. It should be dictated and transcribed within 24 hours of admission and, according to JCAHO and Hillcrest regulations, must be *charted* (placed in the medical record) before surgery can be accomplished. Model Report Form 1 on pages 16–17 displays a model report form for an H&P.

Radiology Report

Radiology is that branch of the health sciences dealing with radioactive substances and radiant energy together with the diagnosis and treatment of disease by means of roentgen rays (x-rays) or ultrasound techniques. The radiology report is a description of the findings and the interpretation of radiographs and other studies done by a radiologist.

Roentgenography is the making of a record of the internal structures of the body by passage of x-rays through the body to act on specially sensitized film. Special studies of the internal organs may require the use of contrast media (dyes) taken orally or by injection. Contrast media may be radiolucent (permitting the passage of roentgen rays) or radiopaque (not penetrable by roentgen rays or other forms of radiant energy). Ultrasonics deals with the frequency range beyond the upper limit of perception by the human ear. Ultrasound is used both therapeutically and as a diagnostic aid.

The numbering of these reports is done sequentially and includes the year performed. For example, a chest film from June 30, 2003, might be numbered 03-9062 to show that 9062 x-rays had been done by that date. Model Report Form 2 on page 18 shows a model radiology report.

Operative Report

Immediately after completion of a surgical procedure, a record of the procedure must be dictated by the physician, transcribed, and placed in the patient's file. This information is necessary for other physicians and allied health professionals who may be attending the patient. Preoperative and postoperative diagnoses are included. The body of the report (findings and procedures) is dictated in narrative form and contains information about the condition of the patient after surgery. See Model Report Form 3 on page 19 for a model operative report.

Pathology Report

Pathology is that branch of medicine dealing with the study of disease. It is divided into anatomic pathology and clinical pathology. Anatomic pathology is the branch of pathology from which tissue reports are issued. The tissue is described both grossly and microscopically by a pathologist, a physician who determines the nature and extent of disease. The gross description of the tissue is done with the naked eye before the tissue is prepared for microscopic study. The microscopic description is done after the tissue has been specially prepared and mounted on a glass slide. It is carefully examined under a microscope, and a final diagnosis is issued. Special stains and other procedures, including consultations, are sometimes necessary to make a final diagnosis.

At Hillcrest these reports are numbered sequentially and include the year performed and a letter to indicate autopsy (A), surgical pathology (S), or cytology report (C). For example, an autopsy done on June 30, 2003, might be numbered 03-A-25 to show that 25 autopsies had been done by that date. Model Report Form 4 on page 20 shows a model pathology report.

Request for Consultation

Consults from physicians specializing in different fields of medicine are necessary to provide proper care for the patient; however, the admitting/attending physician is in charge and maintains continuity of care at all times. For instance, when a patient is admitted to Hillcrest by a medical doctor who later determines that surgery may be necessary, the medical doctor often issues a request for consultation from a surgeon. The chosen surgeon answers this request by examining the patient and dictating a complete report of the examination, including a plan for treatment or surgery, and a prognosis. A model request for consultation form is shown in Model Report Form 5 on pages 21–22.

Discharge Summary

A discharge summary (also called a clinical résumé or final progress note) is required for each patient who is discharged from the hospital. It contains some of the same information that is included in the patient's admission history and physical examination. It also includes information about the admitting diagnosis, surgical procedures performed, laboratory and radiology studies, consultations, hospital course, the condition of the patient at the time of discharge, the medications prescribed on discharge, instructions for continuing care and therapy, prognosis, a discharge diagnosis, and possibly a date for a follow-up office visit. See Model Report Form 6 on pages 23–24 for an example of a discharge summary.

Death Summary

If a patient expires instead of being discharged from Hillcrest, a death summary is dictated. A death summary is a standard medical report *exactly like a discharge summary* but with some important, obvious differences.

The time and date of death, for example, must be recorded. Also included in the death summary might be whether the patient's family agreed to an autopsy, whether the patient had a living will that called for no aggressive therapy, sometimes referred to as "do not resuscitate" or DNR status. Even if a patient does not have a living will, this decision is often made by the family or next of kin in an irreversible situation, and this information would be included in the death summary.

The cause of death may or may not be known when the death summary is dictated. At times, a pending surgical pathology report or autopsy report is needed before the cause of death can be confirmed. A model report form for a death summary is shown in Model Report Form 7 on pages 25–26.

Autopsy Report

An autopsy is done at Hillcrest only with permission from the relatives of the deceased unless the patient has died within 24 hours of admission, has died of an unknown cause, or has died under suspicious circumstances. If a patient case is determined to be medicolegal, that is, pertaining to medicine and the law (or to forensic medicine), the medical examiner or an appointed assistant is in charge of the disposition of the body. Nursing personnel, information management personnel, and physicians on the staff of Hillcrest Medical Center are familiar with the requirements of the medical examiner's office.

The complete autopsy (or necropsy) report includes the following.

1. Preliminary diagnosis
2. Clinical history or brief résumé of the patient's medical history including the course in the hospital
3. Gross examination of the body, both external and internal, including evidence of injury

4. After the tissues removed at autopsy have been prepared, a microscopic description of the diseased organs is dictated along with the final diagnoses. Other special studies, opinions, or summary information may be included in the complete autopsy report depending on the specific nature of the case. See Model Report Form 8 on pages 27–34 for a model autopsy report.

Outpatient Model Reports

The outpatient medical records dictated in the Quali-Care Clinic include many of the same formats used in inpatient medical records, e.g., consults, operative procedures, radiology procedures, and specialty procedures. In addition are the subjective, objective, assessment, plan (SOAP) format; the history, physical, impression, plan (HPIP) format; and correspondence. SOAP and HPIP formats, as well as a sample of correspondence, are included in the model report forms.

Model Report Forms

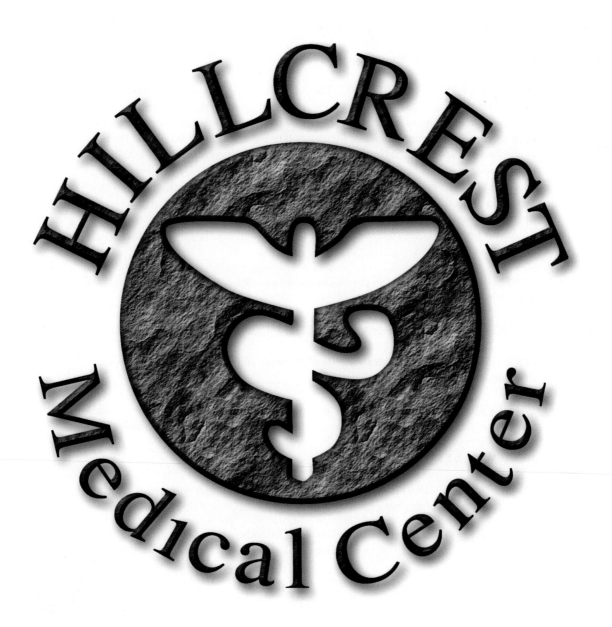

Model Report Form 1

HISTORY AND PHYSICAL EXAMINATION (H&P)

Patient Name: Roger Parks ←————————— 2 spaces after colons
Avoid hyphenation
Hospital No.: 11009   1-inch margins
Left justification

Room No.: 812

Date of Admission: 12/01/- - - - ←————— Format date as MM/DD/YYYY

Admitting Physician: Steven Benard, MD

Admitting Diagnosis: Rule out appendicitis.

CHIEF COMPLAINT: Abdominal pain.

HISTORY OF PRESENT ILLNESS: The patient is a 31-year-old white man with acute onset of right lower quadrant pain waking him up from sleep at approximately 3 a.m. on the morning of admission. The pain worsened throughout the day, radiating to his back and becoming associated with dry heaves. The patient states that the pain is constant and is worsened by walking or movement. The patient states his last bowel movement was on the previous evening and was normal. The patient is anorectic. He also gives a one-year history of lower abdominal colicky pain associated with diarrhea. He was seen by his local medical doctor and given a diagnosis of irritable bowel syndrome; however, the pain is worse tonight and is unlike his previous bouts of abdominal pain. The patient also has had associated fever and chills to date.

PAST HISTORY: Surgical, no previous operations. Illnesses, none. Hospitalized for epididymitis ten years ago.

MEDICATIONS: None. He is ALLERGIC TO PENICILLIN. It makes him bloated.

SOCIAL HISTORY: Carpenter. Lives with his wife and two children. He does not drink or smoke.

FAMILY HISTORY: Insignificant for familial inflammatory bowel disease except for the fact that his mother has colonic polyps. Father living and well. No siblings.

REVIEW OF SYSTEMS: Noncontributory.

PHYSICAL EXAMINATION: This is a 31-year-old white man with knees raised to his abdomen and complaining of severe pain. VITAL SIGNS: Admission

(Continued)   Use colons after brief introducers
First word after a colon begins with a capital letter

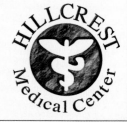

HISTORY AND PHYSICAL EXAMINATION (H&P)
Patient Name: Roger Parks ←———————— **Single space second and**
Hospital No.: 11009   **subsequent page heads**
Date of Admission: 12/01/- - - -
Page 2

←———————————— **Quadruple space between page header and text**
                                below (Text begins on fourth line following head)

temperature 99.6F; four hours after admission it was 102.6F. HEENT:
Normocephalic, atraumatic, EOMs intact, negative icterus, conjunctivae pink.
NECK: Supple. No adenopathy or bruits noted. CHEST: Clear to auscultation and
percussion. CARDIAC: Regular rate and rhythm. No murmurs noted. Peripheral
pulses 2+ and symmetrical. ABDOMEN: Bowel sounds initially positive but
diminished. He has positive cough reflex, positive heel tap, and positive rebound
tenderness. The pain is definitely worse in his RLQ. RECTAL: Heme negative.
Tenderness toward the RLQ. Normal prostate. Normal male genitalia.
EXTREMITIES: No clubbing, cyanosis, or edema. NEUROLOGIC: Nonfocal.

DIAGNOSTIC DATA: Hemoglobin 14.6, hematocrit 43.6, and 13,000 WBCs.
Sodium 138, potassium 3.8, chloride 105, CO_2 24, BUN 10, creatinine 0.9, and
glucose 102. Amylase was 30. UA completely negative. LFTs within normal limits.
Alkaline phosphatase 78, GGT 9, AST 39, GPT 12, bilirubin 0.9. Flat plate and
upright films of the abdomen revealed localized abnormal gas pattern in right lower
quadrant. No evidence of free air.

ASSESSMENT: Rule out appendicitis. Some concern of whether this could be an
exacerbation of developing inflammatory bowel disease. Due to the patient's history,
increasing temperature, and localizing symptoms to his right lower quadrant, the
patient needs surgical intervention to rule out appendicitis.

←———————————— **Quadruple space between last**
No extra space between   **paragraph and signature rule**
dictator/transcriptionist initials

_____ ←—— **Align signature block at left margin;**
Steven Benard, MD   **signature rule is 25 underscores**

                    ←—— **Double space from signature block**
SB:xx   **to dictator/transcriptionist initials***
D:12/01/- - - -
T:12/01/- - - - ←——— **Format dates as MM/DD/YYYY**

*Use either all caps or all lower case for the initials.

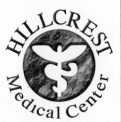

Model Report Form 2

RADIOLOGY REPORT

Patient Name: Marietta Mosley

Hospital No.: 11446

X-ray No.: 03-2801

Admitting Physician: John Youngblood, MD

Procedure: Left hip x-ray.

Date: 08/05/- - - - ←— **Format date as MM/DD/YYYY**

Use 1-inch margins on sides and bottom of report

Use left justification and avoid hyphenation

PRIMARY DIAGNOSIS: Fractured left hip.

CLINICAL INFORMATION: Left hip pain. No known allergies.

Orthopedic device is noted transfixing the left femoral neck. I have no old films available for comparison. The left femoral neck region appears anatomically aligned. At the level of an orthopedic screw along the lateral aspect of the femoral neck, approximately at the level of the lesser trochanter, there is a radiolucent band consistent with a fracture of indeterminate age that shows probable nonunion. There is bilateral marginal sclerosis and moderate offset and angulation at this site.

←————————————— **Double space between paragraphs**

Fairly exuberant callus formation is noted laterally along the femoral shaft.

IMPRESSION
1. No evidence for significant displacement at the femoral neck.
2. Probable nonunion of fracture transversely through the shaft of the femur at about the level of the lesser trochanter.   ←——— **Align text at left margin**

←————— **Quadruple space between last paragraph and signature rule**

_____   **Align signature block with indent command at left**
Neil Nofsinger, MD   ←—   **margin; signature rule is 25 underscores**

←——— **Double space between signature block and**
NN:xx   ←   **dictator/transcriptionist initials**
D:08/05/- - - -   **Transcriptionist's initials (use either all caps**
T:08/05/- - - -   **or all lowercase)**

C: John Youngblood, MD   ←—   **The primary care provider and/or admitting physician gets a copy of medical reports or letters whether or not the name is dictated**

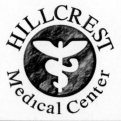

Model Report Form 3

OPERATIVE REPORT

Patient Name: Kathy Sullivan

Hospital No.: 11525

Date of Surgery: 06/25/- - - -

Admitting Physician: Taylor Withers, MD

Surgeons: Sang Lee, MD
Taylor Withers, MD

Preoperative Diagnosis: Urinary incontinence secondary to cystourethrocele.

Postoperative Diagnosis: Urinary incontinence secondary to cystourethrocele.

Operative Procedure: Total abdominal hysterectomy with Marshall-Marchetti correction.

Anesthesia: General endotracheal.

DESCRIPTION: After an abdominal hysterectomy had been performed by Dr. Withers, the peritoneum was closed by him and the procedure was turned over to me.

At this time the supravesical space was entered. The anterior portions of the bladder and urethra were dissected free by blunt and sharp dissection. Bleeders were clamped and electrocoagulated as they were encountered. A wedge of the overlying periosteum was taken and roughened with a bone rasp. The urethra was then attached to the overlying symphysis by placing two No. 1 catgut sutures on each side of the urethra and one in the bladder neck. The urethra and bladder neck pulled up to the overlying symphysis bone very easily with no tension on the sutures. Bleeding was controlled by pulling the bladder neck up to the bone. Penrose drains were placed on each side of the vesical gutter. Blood loss was negligible. The procedure was then turned back over to Dr. Withers, who proceeded with closure.

Sang Lee, MD

SL:xx
D:06/25/- - - -
T:06/26/- - - -

C: Taylor Withers, MD

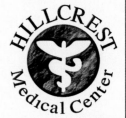

Model Report Form 4

PATHOLOGY REPORT

Patient Name: Sumio Yukimura

Hospital No.: 11449

Pathology Report No.: 03-S-942

Admitting Physician: Donna Yates, MD

Preoperative Diagnosis: Cholelithiasis.

Postoperative Diagnosis: Cholelithiasis.

Specimen Submitted: Gallbladder and stone.

Date Received: 06/05/- - - -

Date Reported: 06/06/- - - -

GROSS DESCRIPTION: Specimen received in one container labeled "gallbladder." Specimen consists of a 9-cm gallbladder measuring 2 cm in average diameter. The serosal surface demonstrates diffuse fibrous adhesion. The wall is thickened and hemorrhagic. The mucosa is eroded, and there is a single large stone measuring 2 cm in diameter within the lumen. Representative sections are submitted in one cassette.

GROSS DIAGNOSIS: Gallstone.

KM:xx
D:06/05/- - - -
T:06/05/- - - -

                **Double space above
and below sign-off
block occurring
between parts of
a report**

MICROSCOPIC DIAGNOSIS: Gallbladder, hemorrhagic chronic cholecystitis with cholelithiasis.

_____
Robert Thompson, MD

RT:xx
D:06/06/- - - -
T:06/06/- - - -

C: Donna Yates, MD

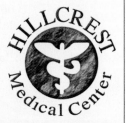

Model Report Form 5

REQUEST FOR CONSULTATION

Patient Name: Marty Gibbs

Hospital No.: 11532

Consultant: Patrick O'Neill, MD, Plastic Surgery

Requesting Physician: Diane Houston, MD, Internal Medicine

Date: 11/25/- - - -

Reason for Consultation: Please evaluate extent of burn injuries.

BURNING AGENT: Coals in fire pit.

I have been asked to see this 5-year-old Caucasian male who appears in mild distress due to upper extremity burn after having fallen into hot coals in his backyard.

Using the Lund Browder chart,[2] the severity of burn is first and second degree. The total body surface area burned includes right lower arm 3%, right hand 1%. The joints involved include the right elbow, right wrist, right hand.

TREATMENT PLAN
Splinting right hand.
Positioning: Elevation with splint on.
Range of motion: Good mobility.
Pressure therapy: Will follow for induration, for pressure fracture.

GOALS
1. Reduce risk of contractures of involved joints by positioning, splinting, and maintaining range of motion.
2. Reduce scar tissue formation by using Jobst bandages, pressure therapy, and splinting.
3. Obtain maximum mobility and strength of upper extremities.
4. Maximize independence in activities of daily living. Activity as tolerated.
5. Provide patient and family education regarding high-calorie, high-protein diet.

←——————————— **Double space above Continued notation**

(Continued)

[2]*See page 197: The Lund Browder Chart.*

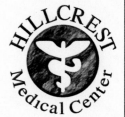

REQUEST FOR CONSULTATION
Patient Name: Marty Gibbs
Hospital No.: 11532
Date: 11/25/- - - -
Page 2

**Single space second and
subsequent page heads**

Thank you for asking me to see this delightful boy. I will follow him at the burn
clinic in two weeks.

_____
Patrick O'Neill, MD

**Include at least two lines of text on the
top of a page with a signature block**

PO:xx
D:11/25/- - - -
T:11/28/- - - -

C: Diane Houston, MD

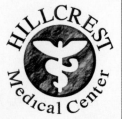

Model Report Form 6

DISCHARGE SUMMARY

Patient Name: Joyce Mabry

Hospital No.: 11709

Admitted: 02/18/- - - -

Discharged: 02/24/- - - -

Consultations: Tom Moore, MD, Hematology

Procedures: Splenectomy.

Complications: None.

Admitting Diagnosis: Elective splenectomy for idiopathic thrombocytopenic purpura and systemic lupus erythematosus.

HISTORY: The patient is a 21-year-old white woman who had noted excessive bruising since last June. She was diagnosed as having thrombocytopenic purpura. At the same time, the diagnosis of systemic lupus erythematosus was made. The patient continues with the bruising. The patient had been treated with steroids, prednisone 20 mg; however, the platelet count has remained low, less than 20,000. The patient was admitted for elective splenectomy.

DIAGNOSTIC DATA ON ADMISSION: Chest x-ray was negative. Electrocardiogram was normal. Sodium 138, potassium 5.2, chloride 104, CO_2 25, glucose 111. Urinalysis negative. Hemoglobin 14.8, hematocrit 43.5, white blood cell count 15,000, platelet count 17,000. PT 11.5, PTT 27.

HOSPITAL COURSE: The patient was taken to the operating room on February 19 where a splenectomy was performed. The patient's postoperative course was uncomplicated with the wound healing well. The platelet count was stable for the first three postoperative days. The patient was transfused intraoperatively with ten units of platelets and postoperatively with ten additional units of platelets. However, on the fourth postoperative day the platelet count had risen to 77,000, which was a significant increase.

The patient was discharged for followup in my office. She will also be seen by Dr. Moore, who will follow her SLE and ITP.

(Continued)

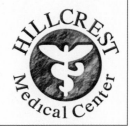

DISCHARGE SUMMARY
Patient Name: Joyce Mabry
Hospital No.: 11709
Discharged: 02/24/- - - -
Page 2

DISCHARGE DIAGNOSES
1. Idiopathic thrombocytopenic purpura.
2. Systemic lupus erythematosus.

DISCHARGE MEDICATIONS ←—————— **No colon used unless words
follow on the same line.**
1. Prednisone 20 mg q.d.
2. Percocet 1 to 2 p.o. q. 4 h. p.r.n.
3. Multivitamins, 1 in a.m. q.d.

_____
Carmen Garcia, MD

CD:xx
D:02/25/- - - -
T:02/26/- - - -

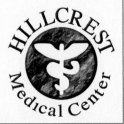

Model Report Form 7

DEATH SUMMARY

Patient Name: Russell Syler

Hospital No.: 11663

Admitted: 05/15/- - - -

Deceased: 06/30/- - - -

Consultations: Hematology/Oncology.

Procedures: Abdominal ultrasound and insertion of Ommaya reservoir.

ADMITTING DIAGNOSES
1. Severe headache pain of two days' duration.
2. Non-Hodgkin lymphoma, large cell type.

FINAL DIAGNOSES
1. Polymicrobial sepsis.
2. Nodular, diffuse, histiocytic lymphoma of head and neck with metastases to central nervous system and liver.
3. Pancytopenia secondary to chemotherapy and sepsis.
4. Bilateral pneumonia.
5. Urinary tract infection due to *Candida* organisms.
6. Oral herpes simplex viral infection.

COURSE IN HOSPITAL: This 33-year-old black man was originally admitted in early April with the diagnosis of nasopharyngeal mixed, nodular, histiocytic, diffuse, large-cell, noncleaved lymphoma with extensive involvement of the paranasal, parapharyngeal, and nasopharyngeal areas with erosion into the left orbit and cribriform plate and possible abdominal involvement. The patient required a tracheostomy secondary to stridor, status post radiation therapy to the neck and face in early May. He was status post chemotherapy with Cytoxan, Adriamycin, vincristine, and prednisone every three weeks. His last chemotherapy had been administered one week prior to the current admission of May 15.

On admission the patient complained of intractable headache pain. He developed fever, chills, and sweats with nausea and vomiting, as well as decreased appetite for at least the past week. He also developed loose bowel movements on the day after admission. He had shortness of breath and a cough productive of yellow phlegm for the past week.

(Continued)

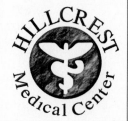

DEATH SUMMARY
Patient Name: Russell Syler
Hospital No.: 11663
Deceased: 06/30/- - - -
Page 2

He had right upper quadrant and epigastric abdominal pain for the past week, not related to meals, with nausea and vomiting. He continued with positive frontal headache as well.

The patient's course deteriorated approximately one week into the hospital course with subsequent hypotension requiring dopamine for maintenance of blood pressure.

DIAGNOSTIC DATA: Blood cultures were positive for *Pseudomonas aeruginosa*. He was treated with tobramycin and penicillin G. As the sensitivity reports were returned from microbiology, vancomycin and Fortaz were added for better *Pseudomonas* coverage. Tobramycin was changed to amikacin when one of the patient's sputum cultures was positive for AFB, atypical, a slow grower, possible *Enterobacter* species.
Two days prior to death, antituberculous medications, including INH and rifampin, were added, as well as amphotericin B for possible systemic fungal infection after urine cultures were positive for *Candida*. He was treated with a five-day course of IV acyclovir for herpes simplex viral infection of the pharynx with resolution of the lesions.

The patient required multiple platelet transfusions as well as packed cells and occasional transfusions of fresh frozen plasma during his admission.

CAUSE OF DEATH: Secondary to circulatory collapse because of overwhelming sepsis, poor immune function, pancytopenia, and diffuse lymphomatous involvement. The patient's wife was notified of the grim prognosis and decided to make the patient "do not resuscitate" status.

The patient was pronounced dead on June 30, - - - -, at 4:12 a.m. Permission for autopsy was requested, but the family refused.

_____

Anthony Zanotti, MD

AZ:xx
D:07/03/- - - -
T:07/05/- - - -

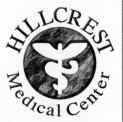

Model Report Form 8

AUTOPSY REPORT

Patient Name: Wayne Kennedy

Hospital No.: 11509

Necropsy No.: 04-A-19

Admitting Physician: Joe Hernandez, MD

Pathologist: Loraine Muir, MD

Date of Death: 04/05/- - - -, 9 p.m.

Date of Autopsy: 04/06/- - - -, 8 a.m.

Admitting Diagnosis: Adenocarcinoma, maxilla.

Prosector: Keith Johnson, PA

FINAL ANATOMIC DIAGNOSES
1. Old fibrotic myocardial infarction of the anterior and septal walls of the left ventricle with anterior ventricular aneurysm, 4.5 x 3.0 cm.
2. Patchy old fibrotic myocardial infarction of the lateral and posterior septal walls of the left ventricle.
3. Probable recent ischemic changes, especially of the anterior and septal walls of the left ventricle.
4. Severe calcified atherosclerotic coronary vascular disease with up to 95% stenosis of the right coronary artery (RCA), up to 70% stenosis of the left anterior descending (LAD) coronary artery, and greater than 95% stenosis of the left circumflex coronary artery (LCCA).
5. Bilateral arterionephrosclerosis.
6. Atherosclerotic vascular disease, aorta, moderate to severe; circle of Willis, moderate.
7. Old infarct of right inner and inferior occipital lobe; small lacunar infarct, right caudate nucleus.
8. Bilateral pulmonary congestion, moderate.
9. Chronic passive congestion, liver, mild.
10. Simple cysts, right and left kidneys, up to 5.5 cm.

(Continued)

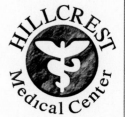

AUTOPSY REPORT
Patient Name: Wayne Kennedy
Hospital No.: 11509
Autopsy: 04/06/- - - -
Page 2

11. Diverticulum, 2.5 cm, duodenum.
12. Diverticulosis, sigmoid colon.
13. Status post partial left maxillectomy for adenocarcinoma, recent.

_____

Loraine Muir, MD

LM:xx
D:04/26/- - - -
T:04/26/- - - -

C: Joe Hernandez, MD

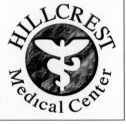

AUTOPSY REPORT

Patient Name: Wayne Kennedy
Hospital No.: 11509
Prosector: Keith Johnson, PA
Assistant: Yang Shen, PA

GROSS AUTOPSY EXAMINATION

CLINICAL SUMMARY: Mr. Kennedy was a 75-year-old married Caucasian man who had been admitted to Hillcrest Medical Center on April 5 for re-resection of a left cheek mass, which had been resected in the past and was reported to be adenocarcinoma with margins involved. (See surgical report No. 03-S-125.) The patient's past medical history was remarkable for coronary artery disease, aortic stenosis, and angina. Past EKG reports revealed right bundle branch block, possible old anterior septal myocardial infarction, and probable ventricular aneurysm. Recent liver function studies were reported to be abnormal.

The patient underwent a partial left maxillectomy on the evening of April 5. The surgical procedure was uneventful, and the patient was sent to PAR in satisfactory condition at 7:55 p.m. However, shortly after his arrival in the recovery room, Mr. Kennedy suffered cardiopulmonary arrest. Code 19 was called at 8:12 p.m., and resuscitation efforts were begun immediately. Despite aggressive efforts, however, the patient was unable to be resuscitated and was pronounced dead at 9 p.m. on April 5.

AUTOPSY PERMISSION: Signed by the wife with no restrictions noted.

TIME AND DATE OF EXAMINATION: April 6, - - - -, 8 a.m.

VISITING PHYSICIANS: None.

EXTERNAL EXAMINATION: The body is that of an adult white man. The external appearance is consistent with the stated age. Total body length is 176 cm. Weight is estimated at 83 kg. The body is identified by a tag. Arterial embalming has not been performed. There is complete rigor mortis. There is posterior dependent lividity. There is moderate cyanosis of the nail beds of the fingers. Body heat and jaundice are absent. The nutritional status is adequate. The hair of the scalp is gray-brown with male pattern baldness. The irides are blue-gray, and the pupils measure 0.6 cm bilaterally. The skin surrounding the left eye has red-purple ecchymotic changes and appears slightly edematous. The sclera of the left eye is moderately congested. There is an 11.5-cm, recently sutured surgical incision beginning just superior to the central aspect of the upper lip and extending along the left side of the nose and beneath the left lower eyelid. An obturator and gauze packing are present in the area of the left maxilla with a portion of the maxilla having been recently surgically resected. An

(Continued)

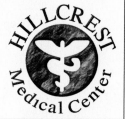

AUTOPSY REPORT
Patient Name: Wayne Kennedy
Hospital No.: 11509
Autopsy: 04/06/- - - -
Page 2

endotracheal tube is in place via the right naris. The ears are unremarkable. The neck is negative for abnormalities. The thoracic wall is normal in symmetry and anteroposterior diameter. A vascular catheter is present in the right subclavian region. The breasts are normal. The abdomen is concave. The external genitalia are normal male. A vascular catheter is present in the posterior aspect of the right hand. Two gold-colored bands are present on the fourth finger of the left hand. There is a rectangular 12.0 x 6.5 cm recent skin graft donor site on the anterior aspect of the left thigh. A 13.5 x 6.5 cm retangular gray-tan to red, apparent previous skin graft donor site is present on the anterior aspect of the right leg. The posterior trunk is unremarkable. There are no palpable lymph nodes. There is no significant peripheral edema.

INCISIONS AND EVISCERATION: The trunk is opened with the usual Y-shaped incision. An intermastoid incision is used for examination of the brain. The organs of the trunk are removed using the Rokitansky method.

SUBCUTANEOUS TISSUE AND MUSCLES: The subcutaneous fat of the midabdomen measures 3 cm in thickness and appears adequately hydrated. The skeletal musculature appears normal.

PERITONEAL CAVITY: The peritoneum is normal. The abdominal organs are normal in relation to each other. There is no increased fluid. There are no adhesions. The diaphragmatic leaves are normal. The inferior hepatic and splenic margins are normally located.

MEDIASTINUM AND THYMUS: The mediastinum is of normal appearance with no shift of the trachea. The thymus is largely replaced by fat.

PLEURAL CAVITIES: There is no increased fluid. There are no adhesions.

PERICARDIAL CAVITY: There is no increased fluid. There are no adhesions.

HEART: The heart weighs 480 g and is normal in size, shape, and position. The epicardial surface is unremarkable. Serial sections through the coronary arteries reveal the proximal 3 cm of the right coronary artery to have approximately 40% to 70% focally calcific atherosclerotic stenosis. An irregular 4.0 x 0.3 x 0.2 cm, tan-red

(Continued)

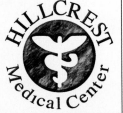

AUTOPSY REPORT
Patient Name: Wayne Kennedy
Hospital No.: 11509
Autopsy: 04/06/- - - -
Page 3

area of discoloration is present within the wall 2 cm from the origin. The subsequent
1.3 cm of the right coronary artery has greater than 95% stenosis with severe
calcification. The remainder of this artery has approximately 20% to 30% stenosis.
The left anterior descending and left circumflex coronary arteries each have separate
ostia arising behind the left cusp of the aortic valve. Each of these ostia is widely
patent. The left anterior descending coronary artery has approximately 40% to 60%
calcific atherosclerotic stenosis throughout its length. The first 2.5 cm of the
circumflex coronary artery has approximately 60% to 75% calcific atherosclerotic
stenosis. A subsequent 0.7-cm segment has tan-red to gray thrombus material filling
its lumen. The subsequent 0.7 cm of this artery has approximately 50% stenosis.
Following this is a 1-cm segment, which is occluded by gray to tan rubbery thrombus
material. The remainder of the artery has approximately 40% to 60% stenosis. A right
dominant coronary arterial system is present. The atria measure 0.2 cm in thickness
and are normal in appearance. The foramen ovale is closed. The right ventricle
measures 0.3 cm in thickness. The left ventricle measures 1.5 cm in thickness just
inferior to the mitral annulus. There is a 4.5 x 3.0 cm soft aneurysmic dilatation of the
central anterior wall of the left ventricle. The anterior wall has transmural gray-white
rubbery fibrotic changes extending from the apex to the central aspect. The wall of
this area ranges in thickness from 0.2 cm to 0.5 cm. There are circumferential rubbery
gray-white fibrotic changes of the apical myocardium of the left ventricle and
transmural, similar fibrotic changes of the septum extending from the apex to the
central portion. In the areas of greatest fibrosis, the septum measures only 0.3 cm in
thickness. Patchy fibrotic changes are present throughout the left half of the remainder
of the septal wall extending to the base. There is slight extension of the fibrotic
changes to the left lateral ventricular wall at the base. There are no mural thrombi.
The endocardium of the aneurysmal area has focal firm gray-tan apparent
calcification, the largest area of which measures 0.1 cm in greatest dimension. The
valves of the heart measure 14, 10, 11, and 7 cm for the tricuspid, pulmonic, mitral,
and aortic, respectively. There is a slight rubbery thickening of the cusps of the aortic
valve, but otherwise the valves are grossly unremarkable. The chordae tendineae and
the trabecular muscle of the right ventricle are multiple, thin, threadlike fibrous bands
that measure less than 0.1 cm in thickness and up to 4.5 cm in length. These bands
form a spiderweb-like meshwork within the right ventricular cavity at the base.

GREAT VESSELS: The main pulmonary arteries contain neither emboli nor
atherosclerotic plaque. The ductus arteriosus is closed. The aorta has moderate to

(Continued)

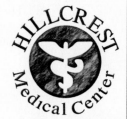

AUTOPSY REPORT
Patient Name: Wayne Kennedy
Hospital No.: 11509
Autopsy: 04/06/- - - -
Page 4

severe calcific atherosclerosis with scattered areas of intimal ulceration measuring up
to 2 cm in greatest dimension. The ostium of the right renal artery has approximately
75% stenosis; the ostium of the left renal artery is widely patent. Both arteries have
mild to moderate atherosclerotic plaque.

THYROID: This gland is normal in shape, size, color, and consistency.

PARATHYROIDS: No enlargement of these glands is demonstrable.

LARYNX AND TRACHEA: The larynx and trachea are normal. There is no
hyperemia of the mucosa.

LUNGS AND BRONCHI: The right lung weighs 520 g. The left lung weighs 420 g.
The pleural surface of each is reddish pink to dark red with mild to moderate
anthracotic pigmentation. The smaller pulmonary arteries contain no emboli or
significant atherosclerotic change. The bronchi contain a small amount of reddish
tan, mucoid-appearing material, and the bronchial mucosa is mildly hyperemic. The
parenchyma of the lower lobes and dependent portions of each lung have a moderate,
dark red, congested appearance. The cut surface exudes a small amount of frothy
pink-red fluid. There is an 0.6 x 0.5 x 0.5 cm, tan, finely granular calcified area
within the parenchyma of the left lower lobe. No other focal lesions are identified. A
lymph node near the hilum of the right lung has an 0.5 cm, firm, calcified, gray
granulomatous-appearing area.

GASTROINTESTINAL TRACT: The esophagus is normal with no significant degree
of leukoplakia. The serosa of the stomach is smooth and glistening. The stomach
contains a small quantity of fluid material. The mucosa of the stomach has the usual
rugal pattern. There are no ulcerations, erosions, or tumors of the gastric mucosa. The
pylorus is normal. There is a 2.5 x 1.5 x 1.5 cm diverticulum of the wall of the
duodenum 8 cm distal to the pyloric sphincter. The ampulla of Vater enters into the
proximal side of this diverticulum. The duodenum is otherwise unremarkable. The small
intestine contains a small amount of liquid material. The mucosa of the small intestine is
normal. The cecum contains a moderate amount of brown semiliquid stool. The mucosa
of the colon is examined in its entirety and found to be normal. No polyps, tumors,
diverticula, or ulcers are noted. The vermiform appendix is unremarkable. The omentum
is normal, as are the mesenteric arteries, veins, and fat.

(Continued)

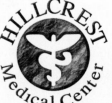

AUTOPSY REPORT
Patient Name: Wayne Kennedy
Hospital No.: 11509
Autopsy: 04/06/- - - -
Page 5

LIVER: The liver weighs 1920 g. The capsule is smooth and glistening with no evidence of thickening. The sectioned surface reveals a normal hepatic parenchyma with no accentuation of the lobular pattern. There are no scars or nodules. The parenchyma is dry and reddish tan. The portal vein and the hepatic artery are normal.

GALLBLADDER: The gallbladder is normal in location, shape, and size and is free of adhesions. It contains a moderate amount of thick, dark green viscid bile. No calculi are present. There are no papillomas of the mucosa, and there is no cholesterolosis. The cystic duct is normal. The common bile duct is somewhat dilated, measuring 2 cm in circumference, but is lined by the usual velvety epithelium. No areas of obstruction are identified.

PANCREAS: The peripancreatic fat is normal. The pancreas is serially sectioned revealing a normal, pale tan, firm consistency. There are no tumor nodules. The pancreatic duct is not distended, and the blood vessels are normal.

SPLEEN: The spleen weighs 140 g. The capsule is smooth and opaque. There are no areas of fibrosis. The sectioned surfaces show no accentuation of the malpighian bodies or trabeculations. The interior of the spleen is dark red and firm.

ADRENALS: These glands are normal in size, shape, consistency, and position. The cortices are a vivid yellow and no nodules are present. The medullae are gray with no nodules.

KIDNEYS: The right kidney weighs 200 g, and the left kidney weighs 210 g. The capsules appear normal and strip with ease. The underlying renal surfaces are dark red and coarsely granular. A large 5.5-cm, smooth-walled cyst filled with straw-colored serous fluid is present in the peripheral cortex of the upper pole of the left kidney. Two similar cysts measuring 3.5 and 2.5 cm in diameter are present within the cortex of the lower pole and central lateral aspect of the right kidney, respectively. The cortices of each kidney range in thickness from 0.4 cm to 0.7 cm. The medullae appear normal. The corticomedullary junctions are mildly indistinct. There are no tumors, infarcts, or areas of scarring. The calyces and pelves are not dilated. The mucosa is normal. The arteries and veins appear normal. The perirenal fat is unremarkable.

URETERS AND BLADDER: The ureters are patent throughout with no dilatations or obstructions. The urinary bladder contains a small amount of yellow urine.

(Continued)

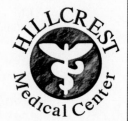

AUTOPSY REPORT
Patient Name: Wayne Kennedy
Hospital No.: 11509
Autopsy: 04/06/- - - -
Page 6

The walls of the bladder are of normal thickness, and the mucosa is moderately trabeculated. No calculi are present within the urinary tract.

GENITAL ORGANS: The prostate is located in the usual position and is normal in size. The parenchyma has the usual gray-pink appearance and rubbery consistency with mild to moderate nodularity. There is no obstruction to the urinary outflow tract. The seminal vesicles are unremarkable. The testicles are normal by palpation.

LYMPH NODES: The right hilar lymph node has the previously described granulomatous area present. Similar, firm, calcified, gray, granulomatous areas are present within two mediastinal lymph nodes, the largest of these granulomatous areas measuring 1.5 cm in greatest dimension. The cervical, periaortic, iliac, mesenteric, omental, and axillary nodes are unremarkable.

BONES AND JOINTS: The cartilage at the sternoclavicular joint is slightly more prominent than usual. The joints otherwise are unremarkable.

BONE MARROW: Vertebral marrow from the lumbar area and from the ribs appears grossly normal.

CRANIAL CAVITY: There is no evidence of recent or old skull fractures, epidural or subdural hemorrhages. There is no focal or diffuse thickening of the skull cap.

BRAIN: The leptomeninges covering the brain are translucent and thin. The brain weighs 1480 g. The gyri and sulci of the cerebral cortex are normal. There are no pressure ridges on the uncinate gyri, and there is no coning of the cerebellum. The vessels comprising the circle of Willis show no abnormalities. No aneurysms are present. There is moderate atherosclerosis. The brain will undergo further fixation in a 10% formalin solution and will be further described at Neuropathology Conference.

_____

Loraine Muir, MD

LM:xx
D:04/06/- - - -
T:04/10/- - - -
←———————————— **Double space between transcribed**
date and copy line
C: Joe Hernandez, MD

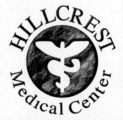

Model Report Form 9

HISTORY, PHYSICAL, IMPRESSION, PLAN (HPIP)

Patient Name: Margaret Thornton
PCP: R. J. Reardon, MD

Date of Birth: 4/7/- - - -   **Age:** 27
Sex: Female

← ———————————— **Double space here and between paragraphs**

Date of Exam: 9/23/- - - -

HISTORY: Fever and some cough since 9/20/- - - - when she was started on Biaxin 500 mg, 1 p.o. b.i.d. Fever has continued since that time at 101.5 Fahrenheit, taken orally as soon as her Tylenol wears off. No current *Pneumocystis* prophylaxis; says that her T-cell count was 86 last time. She complains of headaches but denies changes in vision. She has right-sided chest pain, particularly by the end of the day and with movement. Medications include Mycostatin suspension, multivitamins, Elavil 10 mg p.r.n., Ativan 1 mg b.i.d. p.r.n., the Biaxin, and Diflucan 200 mg, 1 p.o. b.i.d. Only a two-day supply of Diflucan was given. WBC count of 5500 with differential 42% neutrophils, 34% lymphocytes, 9% monocytes, and 3% eosinophils. Hematocrit 44%, platelets 199,000. Chest x-ray: Mild interstitial looking fuzziness bilaterally, more on right than on left.

PHYSICAL EXAMINATION: In general a chronically ill white female, weight down 2 pounds since her last visit, energy level is down. HEENT: Oral cavity erythematous, no thrush. NECK: A few small cervical lymph nodes are palpated. CHEST: Mild decreased breath sounds on the right but no frank rales or rhonchi. No murmurs or rubs. SKIN is clear; no signs of herpes zoster reactivation. Face is somewhat flushed. ABDOMEN is scaphoid with bowel sounds present in all four quadrants. EXTREMITIES: Some mild peripheral neuropathy bilaterally; reflexes and pulses intact bilaterally.

IMPRESSION: Acquired immunodeficiency syndrome with progression of disease.

PLAN: We had a long talk regarding her medication, her T-cell count, the possibility that she has had a progression in her disease, and that she would need to slow down. She is to be off work for this week, and we will see her back here next week.

_____

Robert Solenberger, MD
Infectious Disease

RS:xx
D:9/23/- - - -
T:9/24/- - - -

C: R. J. Reardon, MD

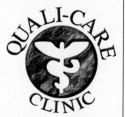

Model Report Form 10

SUBJECTIVE, OBJECTIVE, ASSESSMENT, PLAN (SOAP)

Patient Name: Mitchell Fitzpatrick   **PCP:** Norma Jacobs, MD

Date of Birth: 6/17/- - - -   **Age:** 53   **Sex:** Male

Date of Exam: 2/1/- - - -

SUBJECTIVE
Mr. Fitzpatrick presents for followup of his hemoptysis, which has improved significantly. He underwent flexible fiberoptic bronchoscopy as an outpatient at Hillcrest on 1/27/- - - - with no endobronchial abnormalities noted. It is suspected, therefore, that his expectoration of blood is not coming from his lungs. The patient has had worsening dyspnea on exertion, according to his wife, with several episodes of nocturnal wheezing associated with mild shortness of breath.

OBJECTIVE
Spirometry shows an FEV_1 of 2.59, 82% of predicted. His FEV_1:FVC ratio is 79%. FVC is 3.26, 71% of predicted. There is mild reduction in the midflow rates. On exam, oropharynx is clear. Neck is supple without adenopathy or bruits. Lung fields are clear to auscultation. Cardiac exam: Regular rate and rhythm with a soft systolic murmur heard best at the right upper sternal border and left apex. No significant peripheral edema or cyanosis.

ASSESSMENT
1. Hemoptysis, no evidence of endobronchial lesions.
2. Obesity.
3. Probable bronchospastic lung disease.
4. History of hypertension, remote.
5. History of peptic ulcer disease, remote.

PLAN
1. We will start the patient empirically on an albuterol inhaler, two puffs q. 4 h. p.r.n. wheezing or dyspnea.
2. He will be instructed on the proper use of his inhaler.
3. Followup in four months for repeat spirometry testing.

_____

Gerald Warr Wells, MD
Pulmonology

GWW:xx
D:2/1/- - - -
T:2/2/- - - -

C: Norma Jacobs, MD

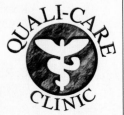

Model Report Form 11

CORRESPONDENCE

QUALI-CARE CLINIC
HEMATOLOGY STE 200
10 MEDICAL BLVD
MIAMI, FLORIDA 33130
Phone: 305/555-2242

June 20, - - - -

Rodney Wells, MD
Florida Center for Infectious Disease
2303 SE Military Dr
Miami, FL 33173

RE: HAL TESCH
        Date of birth: January 24, - - - -

Dear Dr. Wells:

Thank you for the kind referral of your patient, Hal Tesch, regarding his pancytopenia.
He has a history of cirrhosis with portal hypertension. From the information you have
provided me, his pancytopenia was present at the time he presented to your facility on
March 6. His white blood cell count at that time was 3400 with 58 segmented forms.
His WBC count dropped to 2400 on April 4 and was as low as 1900 on June 4. On
June 18 the patient's WBC count was 2300; as we discussed, you gave him Neupogen.
By the next day his WBCs were up to 7400.

Physical examination has revealed evidence of hepatosplenomegaly and chronic liver
disease.

As we discussed, I think the patient's pancytopenia is related to his cirrhosis and
hypersplenism rather than to his antituberculous medications. He had pancytopenia
at essentially the same level as he does now prior to receiving therapy for
tuberculosis. I had planned to get vitamin B_{12}, folate, antinuclear antibody analysis,
and a rheumatoid factor to look for other causes of pancytopenia; however, I suspect
that these studies would be negative. I did not have them drawn in my office but
decided to leave them for you to obtain in your facility, if you feel they are
warranted.

(Continued)

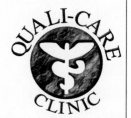

Rodney Wells, MD
June 20, - - - -
RE: Hal Tesch
Page 2

I recommend continuing the patient on Neupogen at 5 mg/kg probably about three times weekly. I found it impressive that he received his first dose of Neupogen on June 18 and by just the next day his white blood cell count had risen from 2300 to 7400.

Thank you for allowing me to participate in the care of this very pleasant gentleman. I will return him to your care, though I would be delighted to see him at any time I can be of further assistance.

Sincerely,

Stephen C. Gordon, MD
Hematology

SCG:xx

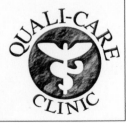

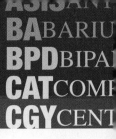

SECTION 3
References

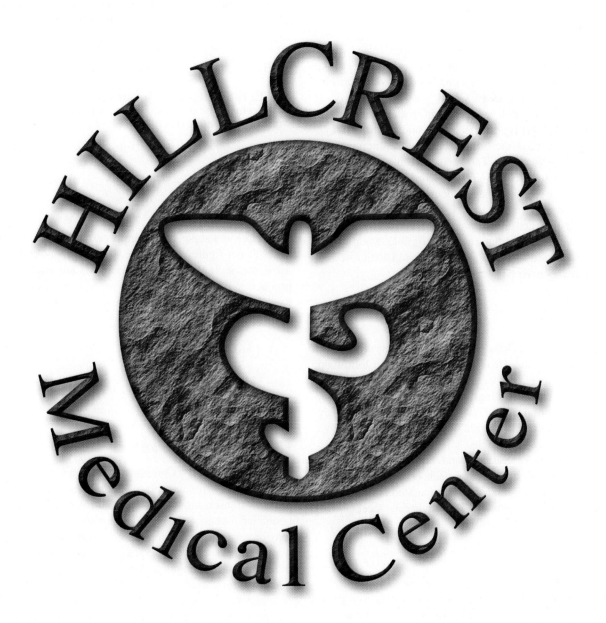

Transcription Rules for Hillcrest Medical Center and Quali-Care Clinic

Each hospital has a process by which the abbreviations and style for its transcribed medical records are set. This process usually involves an information management committee (comprised of appointed members of the medical staff) together with representatives from both the information management department and hospital administration. The rules adopted for medical reports at Hillcrest have been voluntarily adopted for use at Quali-Care Clinic, and they include the following.

Style Variations

Flexibility in medical transcription is important. Doctors employ variations in style when dictating their records, and medical transcriptionists must be able to conform to these styles when necessary. Check for your employer or client preferences and be consistent within each one's body of work. This practice is easily said but not always easily done because the originators may be inconsistent within their own work. The medical transcriptionist is charged with turning the spoken word into the written word, to create not only a legal document but also one that makes the employer or client look good. That is, transcriptionists correct dictation errors in English grammar, usage, and sentence structure when possible. Style variations that you are likely to see used both in Hillcrest and on the job are listed below.

HEADINGS

Headings that stand alone take *no* colon unless words follow on the same line. Headings with words that follow on the same line take a colon, and the first word that follows is uppercase. These headings, however, may be uppercase, may have an initial capital letter, be bold or not bold, may be centered, at the left margin, or tabbed. All of the above heading styles are acceptable.

The Review of Systems and Physical Examination paragraphs may be one paragraph each, or the internal headings within each paragraph may be separated out with each heading beginning a new line. Both styles are acceptable.

LISTS

Lists of medications, diagnoses, procedures, etc., may be indented, tabbed, at the left margin, or all in one paragraph. They may be numbered with the 1, 2, 3 system or with a, b, c. At times you will see (1), (2), (3) or even 1), 2), 3) used. More elaborate lists might use Roman numerals with subheadings. This style is not normally utilized in the transcription of medical records; however, it is as correct as any of the above-listed numbering styles for lists.

DATES

Date styles are either numeric or written in words. Both are acceptable in medical transcription. Use the style as dictated by the originator. See the following examples.

1/1/2004	1 Jan 2004	1 January 2004
01/01/2004	Jan 1, 2004	January 1, 2004

NOTE: Hillcrest is using a four-digit year because the style seems to be going that way. A two-digit year would be just as correct.

Remember, for your work at Hillcrest, use ---- instead of a year.

SUBSCRIPTS AND SUPERSCRIPTS

Subscripts and superscripts can be used, but because it is faster to put figures on the line, some styleguides recommend this style. Many transcriptionists are paid by their production of work, so time is money. (It is possible to put these in AutoText if you want the subscript or superscript without the extra work.)

Examples
S_1, S_2 *or* S1, S2
CO_2 *or* CO2
m^2 *or* sq m

CONTINUED PAGES

At Hillcrest we use "(Continued)" at the end of pages that are continued. In some places of business, however, the medical transcriptionist has no control over this due to computer footers that are added automatically. This style may or may not be able to be used on the job.

Page-two headings are always used in one way or another. An on-the-job computer system may automatically add this information in a header. If not, use your employer or client preference. At Hillcrest we use different page-two headings for inpatient reports, outpatient reports, and correspondence.

SIGNATURE LINE

The signature line at Hillcrest (25 underscores) is placed at the left margin; however, some places tab the signature line to the center of the page. Both styles are acceptable. Remember, in correspondence an actual line is not used for the signature. Just allow four spaces before typing the originator's name. The signature will go in that space.

SIGN-OFF BLOCK

The sign-off block is always used in medical transcription but not necessarily in correspondence. The sign-off block can vary widely in style, so stay flexible. The initials can be all uppercase, all lowercase, or a combination. The dates are usually numeric but can be done in a couple of styles. Hospitals and transcription companies sometimes customize the sign-off block.

COPY LINE

The copy line, which is typed two spaces below the sign-off block, can be C or c (copy), CC or cc (courtesy copy), PC or pc (photocopy). Any one of these styles is acceptable.

ENCLOSURE LINE

If your report or letter includes an enclosure, this information is noted by the word "Enclosure" typed two spaces below the copy line. This can be abbreviated as either Enc. or Encl.

NOTE: At the end of a letter or a report, to keep it from going onto another page, you can adjust the spaces between signature line, sign-off block, copy line, and enclosure line. You may not go to an extra page unless there are at least two lines of type from the body of the report on the new page. (There should be no pages with just a signature line or even less on them.) If you cannot arrange the information to keep it from going onto another page, then place at least two lines of type from the body of the report on the new page.

Capitalization

1. Use initial capital letters in eponymic terms. Eponyms are names of phrases formed from or including the name of a person. The common noun following the eponym is lowercase.

   Examples
   > Rockey-Davis incision
   > Foley catheter
   > Down syndrome
   > May Hegglin anomaly
   > Duffy blood group
   > Crohn's disease

NOTE: Over the past several years there has been a trend away from using the possessive form in eponymic terms. The *AAMT Book of Style* (2nd ed.), *Dorland's Illustrated Medical Dictionary,* and *Stedman's Medical Dictionary* recognize this trend; however, the possessive form is still acceptable if your facility prefers or dictates that style. Both styles appear in this text-workbook.

2. Capitalize trade names and proprietary names of drugs and brand names of manufactured products and equipment. Do *not* capitalize generic names or descriptive terms.

   Examples
   > Trade names of drugs include Keflex, Motrin, and Bayer. Corresponding generic terms are cephalaxin, ibuprofen, and aspirin.
   > Trade names of suture materials include Vicryl, Dexon, and Prolene. Generic terms include chromic catgut, silk, nylon, and cotton—either plain, braided, or twisted.
   > Miscellaneous brand names include Kleenex, Vaseline, and Scotch tape. Corresponding generic terms are tissue, petroleum jelly, and cellophane tape.

3. Use an initial capital letter and italics (or underscore to indicate italics) for the name of a genus when used in the singular. Do not capitalize, italicize, or underscore when used in the plural or as an adjective. See "The Grammar of Microbiology" on page 46.

   Example
   > *Pseudomonas aeruginosa (P. aeruginosa)*
   > **BUT**
   > pseudomonal appearing

4. Departmental names within Hillcrest Medical Center are lowercase.

   Examples
   > operating room
   > postanesthesia recovery
   > blood bank
   > transcription section

5. Capitalize the proper names of languages, races, religions, and sects. Do *not* capitalize the common nouns following these designations. Do *not* capitalize informal designations of race, i.e., white or black.

   Examples
   > Asians
   > Hispanic people
   > the English language
   > of Jewish ancestry

African-Americans
Seminoles

6. As a courtesy, positive allergy information may be either bolded or keyed in all capital letters in order to call attention to this vital information.

Example
ALLERGIES: The patient is allergic to SULFA.

7. Capitalize acronyms but not the words from which the acronym is derived.

Examples
nonsteroidal anti-inflammatory drug (NSAID)
coronary artery bypass graft (CABG)
magnetic resonance imaging (MRI)

Numbers

1. Spell the numbers "one" through "ten" when they appear in a narrative section of a medical report. When one numerical expression follows another, for clarity, spell out the one that can more easily be expressed in words.

Examples
Dr. Smith removed seven lesions from the patient's back and three from his right leg.
The dietician recommended two 6-ounce cans of supplement daily.

2. Use figures with technical information, i.e., in laboratory results, vital signs, age, height, weight, drug dosages.

Examples
Apgar scores were 9 and 9 at one and five minutes. (*AAMT Book of Style*)
Apgar scores were 9/9 at 1 and 5 minutes. (*AMA Manual of Style*)
Lipoproteins included an LDL of 80 and an HDL of 50.
Vital signs showed blood pressure 120/80, pulse 72/minute and regular, respirations 21, temperature 98 degrees F. (See "Vital Signs" on page 45.)
Medications: Lomotil 20 mg at bedtime, diazepam 15 mg daily.

3. Always use figures with abbreviations, symbols, and technical measurements—no space comes between the number and its symbol, but use one space before and after the "x" in measurements.

Examples
Pulses 2+, 100% oxygen, 15 mmHg, reflexes 5/5 throughout

The uterus weighs 150 g and measures 8.0 x 4.5 x 0.9 cm.

NOTE: In the measurement above, while the whole number has a zero added for balance, the final measurement has a preceding zero added for clarity. *The preceding zero is mandatory in decimal phrases.*

4. A space should appear between an Arabic number and the corresponding unit of measure abbreviation/symbol.

Examples
9 mg%, 83 mL, 0.5 cm, 64 g/dL

5. Spell out ordinal numbers *except* when a date is used with the month.

Examples
An incision was made between the fifth and sixth ribs. (*or* 5th and 6th)
The patient had a seventh nerve palsy. (*or* 7th, *not* VIIth)
A Foley catheter was inserted the third day after surgery.

BUT

On October 3 surgery was performed.

6. Numbers that constitute a series or range should be written as figures if at least one of them is greater than ten or is a mixed or decimal fraction. When indicating a span of years or page numbers do *not* omit digits.

Examples
The gallstones measured 0.5 and 3.7 cm, respectively.
Statistics proved the theory in 8 of 12 recipients.
The patient took epilepsy medication from 2000 to 2003 (*not* 2000–03)
The solution can be found on pages 157 through 159. (*not* 157–159)

NOTE: When the phrase "from _____ to _____" is used, the "to" is spelled out. The same is true when the phrase "between _____ and _____" is used. The "and" is spelled out. A hyphen is not used in either of these phrases to avoid unnecessary confusion.

7. The vertebral or spinal column segments are referred to in Arabic numerals. The 12 pairs of cranial nerves, however, are referred to in Roman numerals.

Examples
cervical spine = C1 through C7
thoracic spine = T1 through T12
dorsal spine = D1 through D12
    (interchangeable with thoracic spine)

lumbar spine = L1 through L5
sacral spine = S1 through S5

BUT

cranial nerves I through XII

8. Titers and ratios are expressed with figures and a colon. The colon is read as "to."

   Examples
   Cord blood sample showed a herpes titer of 1:110.
   Anesthesia consisted of Xylocaine and epinephrine 1:100,000.

9. Temperature readings are expressed in either Celsius (C) or Fahrenheit (F). At Hillcrest, the symbol for the word "degrees" is not used.

   Each of the following examples is acceptable.

   98.6F or 98.6 degrees Fahrenheit

   35.4C or 35.4 degrees Celsius

10. Stainless and nonstainless steel sutures are sized by the United States Pharmacopeia (USP) system. Sizes range from 11-0 (smallest) to 7 (largest). Sizes No. 1 through No. 7 are expressed as whole numbers. Stainless steel suture sizes may also be sized by the Brown and Sharp (B&S) gauge. B&S sizes are expressed in whole numbers from No. 40 (smallest) to No. 20 (largest).

    Examples
    Then 9-0 silk was used for the eye wounds.
    The peritoneum was closed with 3-0 chromic catgut.
    No. 5 wire was used for the skin.

    NOTE: In the previous example, "No. 5" is the preferred style for Hillcrest, though "#5" is equally correct except at the beginning of a sentence.

11. Superscripts and subscripts are used in medical dictation; however, if the transcription equipment being used does not provide for entering characters either above or below the line, the superscript and/or subscript may be entered on the line. In either case, no spaces should be used.

    Examples

H2O or H_2O		PO2 or PO_2
$1^3$1I	**BUT**	I 131
$1^2$8 Au	**BUT**	Au 198

12. Use Arabic numerals when referring to EKG leads, cancer grades, and both conventional and military time.

    Examples
    EKG leads V1 to V6   grade 2 tumor
    1600 hours is 4 p.m.

**NOTE: When time on a clock is used to describe a location, use the following style.
Suspicious area was tagged with a suture at 3 o'clock.
Lesions identified at 12, 3, and 6 o'clock.**

Punctuation

APOSTROPHE

1. The apostrophe is used to show possession.

   Examples
   Patient's condition (singular possessive noun)
   Doctors' opinion (plural possessive noun)

2. The apostrophe is used to form contractions, but use contractions only in direct quotes.

   Examples
   He's having no symptoms. (contraction of he is)
   It's my opinion. (contraction of it is)
   BUT
   Its measurements are irregular. (possessive pronoun—no apostrophe used here)

3. Do *not* use an apostrophe to form the plural of either an all-capital abbreviation or of numerals, including years.

   Examples
   DRGs   Temperature in the 20s
   WBCs   Born in the 1990s
   D&Cs   Three PhDs attended

   NOTE: When a word or letter could be misread, the apostrophe is sometimes used for clarity.

   Examples

He received all A's.	The T's were left uncrossed.
Her U's need work.	Record the patient's I's and O's.

4. The apostrophe is used with units of time and money when used as possessive adjectives.

   Examples
   a week's work/a dollar's work/in a month's time (all show singular possessive)
   seven days' work/50 cents' worth/six months' gestation (all show plural possessive)

HYPHEN

1. Hyphenate a compound in which a number is the first element and the compound precedes the noun it modifies.

Examples

48-hour turnaround   a 12-factor panel
a 5-g cyst   two 6-inch lacerations

2. Hyphenate a compound adjectival phrase when it precedes the noun it modifies, but *not* when it is in the predicate.

Examples

a 17-week infant (The infant was 17 weeks old.)
end-to-end anastomosis (The anastomosis was end to end.)
a figure-of-eight suture (The suture was in a figure of eight.)

3. Hyphenate an adjective-noun compound when it precedes and modifies another noun.

Examples

upper-range results (The results were in the upper range.)
third-floor burn unit (The burn unit was on the third floor.)

4. Hyphenate two or more adjectives used coordinately or as conflicting terms whether they precede the noun or follow as a predicate adjective.

Examples

false-positive results (The results were false-positive.)
double-blind study (The study was done as a double-blind.)

5. Hyphenate color terms when the two elements are of equal weight.

Examples

pink-tan tissue   gray-brown area
BUT
pinkish tan mucosa   grayish brown skin

6. When expressing numbers in words, hyphenate all compound numbers between 21 and 99, either ordinal or cardinal numbers. Also, use a hyphen when expressing fractions in words.

Examples

thirty-five miles later
one hundred forty-five
left one-third empty
three-fourths agreed

7. Use a hyphen when joining numbers or letters to form a word, phrase, or abbreviation.

Examples

5-FU   C-section   X-ray   T-spine
VP-16   SMA-12   Y-shaped incision

Abbreviations and Symbols

ABBREVIATIONS

Abbreviations used in Hillcrest Medical Center case studies are listed and defined in the medical terminology glossary preceding each case. They are also listed alphabetically in the index.

"Abbreviations are a convenience, a time saver, a space saver, and a way of avoiding the possibility of misspelling words. However, a price can be paid for their use. Abbreviations are sometimes not understood, misread, or are interpreted incorrectly. Their use may lengthen the time needed to train individuals in the health fields, wastes the time of healthcare workers in tracking down their meaning, at times delays the patient's care, and occasionally results in patient harm.

"Healthcare organizations are wisely required by the Joint Commission on Accreditation of Healthcare Organizations to formulate an approved list of abbreviations. Every attempt should be made to restrict this list to common abbreviations that are understood by all health professionals who must work with medical records."[3]

The information presented in both the heading of each Hillcrest medical report and, at times, in the body of the report will be in what is known as elliptical or "clipped" expressions, i.e., a word or words that represent a complete thought. These clipped expressions are commonly used in medical dictation and each will end with a period to show they are complete thoughts.

NOTE: Hillcrest medical records will have no abbreviations used in the diagnosis lines, impression lines, preoperative or postoperative lines.

SYMBOLS

1. The virgule (slash or diagonal) is used to indicate the word "per" in laboratory values and other equations or the word "over" in blood pressure (BP) readings and visual acuity.

Examples

using the virgule for "per"
hemoglobin 14.1 g/dL
fasting blood sugar 138 mg/dL
using the virgule for "over"
blood pressure 110/70 mmHg in both arms
20/80 right eye and 20/40 left eye (visual acuity)

[3]*Reprinted with permission from* Medical Abbreviations: 12,000 Conveniences at the Expense of Communications and Safety, *11th edition, 2003, published by Neil M. Davis Associates, Huntingdon Valley, Pennsylvania 19006.*

NOTE: When millimeters of mercury is dictated with a blood pressure reading or ocular tension, transcribe mmHg. (Leave out the word "of.")

2. Lowercase x is used to indicate "by" in measurements, to indicate "times" in magnification and multiplication, and to indicate "for" in other phrases. If the x can be read as the word "for," then use the word, not "times" and not x.

   Examples

   Sponge and instrument count was correct x3.
   Electron microscopy cells are magnified x100,000.
   (x = times; no space is left between the x and the number; do not separate at the end of a line)
   Fetal limb length was 5.5 x 1.5 x 1.0 cm.
   (x = by; leave a space both before and after the x; can be separated at the end of a line)
   Dictated: Medication is to be taken *times* six months.
   Transcribed: Medication is to be taken *for* six months.

3. Use numerals with a symbol or an abbreviation. When the phrase is spelled out, however, spell out the number as well.

   Examples

   Deep tendon reflexes two plus (not two +)
   OR
   Deep tendon reflexes 2+ (not 2 plus)

4. Both reflexes and pulses are usually graded on a scale from zero to four plus. The meanings of the different grades are as follows.
   Reflexes
   4+ = very brisk, hyperactive; may indicate disease; often associated with clonus (alternating muscular contraction and relaxation in rapid succession)
   3+ = brisker than average; possibly but not necessarily indicative of disease
   2+ = average or normal
   1+ = somewhat diminished; low normal
   0 = no response; may indicate neuropathy
   Pulses
   0 = completely absent
   +1 = markedly impaired
   +2 = moderately impaired
   +3 = slightly impaired
   +4 = normal

5. Qualitative test results are usually given using the plus and minus symbols.

   Examples

   − negative
   +/− very slight trace or reaction
   + slight trace or reaction
   ++ trace or noticeable reaction
   +++ moderate amount of reaction
   ++++ large amount of pronounced reaction

6. The metric system of measurement is used in medicine. (See the list that follows.) Use the abbreviated forms when entering a number with metric measurements. Do not use a period following metric abbreviations. Do not pluralize abbreviations. (Liter is abbreviated with an uppercase L.)

   Examples

1 cm	0.9 cm	20 cm
1 mL	1.6 mL	15 mL
1 g	3.7 g	32 g
1 L	2.5 L	8 L

7. Latin abbreviations: At Hillcrest these are keyed in lowercase with periods as follows.
   a.c. (ante cibum, before meals)
   a.d. (auris dextra, right ear)
   a.m. (ante meridiem, morning)
   a.s. (auris sinistra, left ear)
   a.u. (auris utraque, each ear)
   b.i.d. (bis in die, twice a day)
   d. (die, day)
   h. (hour)
   h.s. (hora somni, bedtime)
   n.p.o. (nil per os, nothing by mouth)
   o.d. (oculus dexter, right eye)
   o.s. (oculus sinister, left eye)
   o.u. (oculus uterque, each eye)
   p.c. (post cibum, after meals)
   p.m. (post meridiem, afternoon)
   p.o. (per os, by mouth)
   p.r.n. (pro re nata, as circumstances may require)
   q.d. (quaque die, every day)
   q.h. (quaque hora, every hour)
   q.i.d. (quater in die, four times a day)
   q.l. (quantum libet, as much as desired)
   q.p. (quantum placeat, as much as desired)
   q.s. (quantum satis, sufficient quantity)
   t.i.d. (ter in die, three times a day)

List of Metric Measurements

Unit	Abbreviation
centimeter(s)	cm
cubic centimeter(s)	cc or cm^3
cubic meter(s)	m^3
deciliter(s)	dL
gram(s)	g
kilocalorie(s)	kcal
kilogram(s)	kg
kiloliter(s)	kL
kilometer(s)	km
liter(s)	L
meter(s)	m
microgram(s)	mcg
milligram(s)	mg
milliliter(s)	mL
millimeter(s)	mm
square centimeter(s)	sq cm or cm^2
square kilometer(s)	sq km or km^2
square meter(s)	sq m or m^2

The Grammar of Microbiology

Microbiology is a fascinating field of knowledge about which transcriptionists seldom get to be experts. Here are some tips to remember for accuracy.

1. Only when the full genus and species names are used is the phrase italicized.

2. In handwriting or on a keyboard an underscore indicates italics. Because of the italics feature on computers, the underline is seldom used in this manner; however, underlining a genus and species still indicates italics to a typesetter.

3. When the full genus and species names are used, the genus takes an initial cap. When the genus is referred to as a single letter, that letter is uppercase.

4. When medical jargon or slang is dictated, try to transcribe at least the short form except as noted (see following table for usage).

Genus and Species	Short Form	Jargon or Slang Sometimes Dictated	Disease Examples
Branhamella catarrhalis	*B. catarrhalis*	B. cat	otitis media, URIs
Clostridium difficile	*C. difficile**	C. diff	enterocolitis
Coccidioides immitis	*C. immitis*	cox	coccidioidomycosis
Escherichia coli	*E. coli*	—	UTIs, diarrhea
Haemophilus influenzae	*H. influenzae*	H. flu	epiglottitis, pneumonia
Haemophilus vaginalis	*H. vaginalis*	H. vag	vaginal infections
Helicobacter pylori	*H. pylori*	H. py	gastric ulcers
Klebsiella pneumoniae	*K. pneumoniae*	K. pneumo	bacterial pneumonia
Mycobacterium avium-intracellulare	*M. avium-intracellulare*	MAI**	pulmonary disease
Staphylococcus aureus	*S. aureus*	MRSA**	methicillin-resistant staph aureus
Staphylococcus epidermidis	*S. epidermidis*	staph epi or MRSE**	peritonitis, endocarditis, methicillin-resistant staph epidermidis
Staphylococcus pyogenes	*S. pyogenes*	staph pyo	impetigo, scalded skin syndrome
Streptococcus pneumoniae	*S. pneumoniae*	strep pneumo	lobar pneumonia
Streptococcus pyogenes	*S. pyogenes*	strep pyo	septic sore throat, scarlet fever, rheumatic fever

The species "difficile" is correctly pronounced "dif fi' cil ee." We are used to hearing "dif fa ceel"; however, if you hear the first pronunciation, please know what is being dictated.

**MAI, MRSA, and MRSE are common abbreviations, well recognized in medicine. Do not change these abbreviations, if dictated.

Vital Signs

In the following eight dictated vital signs, you will note different sequences *and* different criteria, even though these doctors practice in the same clinic setting. Each doctor dictates patients' vital signs in the same sequence, sometimes dictating the numbers only without using words.

Dictated Vital Signs	Originator's Initials
1. Blood pressure, pulse, respirations, temperature BP 120/80, P 79, R 22, T 98	SCC
2. Temperature, pulse, blood pressure T 99, P 82, BP 156/90	DHG
3. Blood pressure, pulse, temperature, weight BP 90/70, P 65, T 100.1, weight 102-1/2 pounds	REB
4. Temperature, pulse, blood pressure, weight T 95.5, P 82, BP 140/75, weight 190-3/4 pounds	TDF
5. Weight, blood pressure, temperature, pulse Weight 264 pounds, BP 200/100, T 99.6, P 102	JAL
6. Blood pressure, temperature, pulse, respirations BP 132/78, T 97.5, P 72, R 20	JEM
7. Temperature, blood pressure, weight, height T 98.7, BP 145/69, weight 156 pounds, height 63 inches	STW
8. Blood pressure alone BP 179/83	JDMc

Future physicians begin dictating patient records early in their training and might copy a mentor, a fellow student, or just do what comes naturally. No one teaches them exactly how to dictate their records. It is the medical transcriptionists' job to transcribe each originator's dictation correctly and in the originator's specific style.

In the previous eight examples, the transcriptionist should *not* make the styles the same and *not* add information that was not dictated. If the dictation is cut off or unclear, leave a blank and/or flag the report for the originator. If you have access to the medical record, you may look up the vitals and include the correct information. Check the date of visit *and* the date of dictation to get the correct numbers for the record.

Difficult Singular and Plural Words and Phrases

The following words have proven to be difficult because you cannot rely on their being dictated correctly. *Beware* and transcribe as follows.

Singular	Plural
ala nasi is	alae nasi are
diverticulum is	diverticula are
genitalis is	genitalia are
naris is	nares are
medium is	media are
labium	labia
majus is	majora are
minus is	minora are
lentigo is	lentigines are
focus is	foci are
fossa is	fossae are
decubitus *ulcer* is	decubitus *ulcers* are

NOTE: Decubitus is *not* a noun and has no plural form.

Temperature versus Fever

If a dictator says "Patient has some headache but no temperature," remember we *always* have a temperature, it just may not be elevated. Correctly transcribed, the phrase should read either, "Patient has some headache but no elevated temperature" or "Patient has some headache but no fever."

A Tongue Twister

The following changes are found in patients with chronic muscle spasm. The difference between chronic spasm and newly acquired spasm can be palpated and may be described as either

> tense, tender tissue texture changes

> **OR**

> tender tissue texture changes

Dermatology Terms

Hair cycles or phases include (1) anagen, (2) catagen, and (3) telogen. Examples include anagen effluvium, a loss of hair after chemotherapy, and telogen effluvium, a loss of hair due to the trauma of surgery, high fever, stress, etc.

pyknotic nuclei = a thickening of the nuclei

arrectores pilorum = muscles in the connective tissue of the upper dermis, attached to the hair follicles below the sebaceous glands

delling = the formation of a slight blister or dimpling

Pulmonary Terms

> I:E ratio (dictated "eye to E")

> The ratio of inspiratory to expiratory time.

> E → A (dictated "E to A")

> When the patient's saying E, E, E comes out as A, A, A upon auscultation of the lung, this shows consolidation of the lung.

Race

When transcribing race, Caucasian and African American are properly capitalized; however, white and black are properly lowercased.

> **Examples**
> This 45-year-old black female . . .
> This 72-year-old white male . . .
> A 15-month-old Caucasian girl . . .
> A 25-year-old black Cuban male . . .
>
> **OR**
>
> This black male patient is 15 years old.
> My Anglo gardener is 74 years old.
> An African-American girl 9 months old . . .
> His boy, a Native American, is 7 years old.

NOTE: "45-year-old" is a single modifier adjective and needs hyphens. "74 years old" does not use hyphens. Clue: If the term is "years," then no hyphen is needed; if the term is "year," then a hyphen is needed.

Age

In age references, remember

- Neonates or newborns are people from birth to 1 month of age.
- Infants are people 1 month to 24 months of age.
- Children are people 2 years to 13 years of age, also boys or girls.
- Adolescents are people 13 to 17 years of age, also teenagers, boys, or girls.
- Adults are people 18 years of age or older, also men or women.

Zero Safety

Preceding zeros with decimals: These are important safety factors in transcription. In either typewritten or handwritten records, a decimal point on the line is hard to see, is easily missed, and incorrect dosing can result. The preceding zero is essential in transcription.

> **Examples**
> Dictated "Xylocaine point 1 percent," should be transcribed: Xylocaine 0.1%.
> A drug dosage dictated as .25 should be transcribed: 0.25.

NOTE: This pertains only to zeros in front of decimals (preceding zeros), and not to those behind the decimal.

Roman Numerals

When Roman numerals are used in dictating the digits, they mean the following.

> I   digitus primus manus = digit I (thumb)
> II digitus secundus manus = digit II (index finger)
> III digitus tertius manus = digit III (long finger)
> IV digitus quartus manus = digit IV (ring finger)
> V   digitus quintus manus = digit V (little finger)

Roman numerals used with proper names take no comma *before* the numeral.

> **Examples**
> Magnus Flaws III, CPA
> Gerald B. Hensley II, MD

NOTE: See "Class and Stage" for more on Roman numerals.

Time

When transcribing time followed by a.m. or p.m., use no zeros and no colon when the full hour is given.

> **Example**
> Take the medication at 8 a.m., noon, and 4 p.m.; however, take a meal at 7:30 a.m., 11:30 a.m., and 3:30 p.m.

When 12 o'clock is specified as *time,* use noon or midnight. No numerals are necessary.

A 50-pack-year smoking history = smoking a pack a day for 50 years. The pack-year is the result of the *packs per day multiplied by the number of years of smoking.*

Abduction versus Adduction

Abduction means moving away from the midline. (To *ab*duct is to take away.) Adduction means moving toward the midline. (To *ad*duct means to draw toward.) These two words are often dictated using letters at the beginning; for example, "a-b duction" or "a-d duction," since it is hard to hear the difference between "ab" and "ad" when spoken.

Class and Stage

Numbers used in the class and stage of disease can vary widely; however, in cancer terminology, class is generally given in Arabic numerals with stage given in Roman numerals. In rheumatoid arthritis terminology, however, both class and stage are given in Roman numerals, for example, stage I (early disease), stage II (moderate disease), stage III (severe disease), and stage IV (terminal). Class I would indicate complete functional capacity, class II adequate functional capacity, class III the ability to perform few to no activities of daily living (ADLs), and class IV an incapacitated patient—either bedridden or confined to a wheelchair.

Connective Tissues

Connective tissues can attach, bind, and/or support.

> **Examples**
> Fascia attaches muscle to muscle.
> Tendons bind muscle to bone.
> Ligaments attach bone to bone.
> Cartilage supports, covers, and provides firmness, but does not connect.

Subjective versus Objective

The review of systems is a subjective examination; that is, the patient describes his or her feelings, symptoms, etc., which the doctor records. The subjective examination, therefore, consists of data reported by the patient. The physical examination is objective; that is, the doctor dictates what he or she sees and feels.

Surgical Terms

SHARP AND BLUNT DISSECTION

The phrase "sharp and blunt dissection" takes a singular verb. The idea is that the surgeon is separating tissues by a process alternately involving *sharp* use of instruments (snipping with scissors or cutting with a scalpel) and *blunt* use (inserting scissors or clamp with blades closed, then opening them to establish a plane of separation; or using a finger, sponge, or instrument to develop a separation already started). Hence the whole process is just one dissection, but it involves two different types of activity. A singular verb is appropriate.

SUTURE SIZING

The Brown & Sharp (B&S) gauge uses whole numbers, ranging from 40 to 20 (smallest to largest), making a size 35 suture smaller than a size 25 suture.

The USP system sizes steel, silk, cotton, and other materials ranging from 11-0 to 7 (smallest to largest). This makes a size 7 suture different from and larger than a size 7-0. Remember, this is a zero, dictated as "seven oh." Use either 0 or 1-0 cotton, 00 or 2-0 silk, 000 or 3-0 Vicryl; however, for >000, use the "digit-zero" style, as in y-0. The many brand names of suture materials will have an initial capital letter (initial cap), and the generic names will be in all lowercase.

Gynecology Terms

Gravida 6, para 4-0-2-3 refers to 6 pregnancies, resulting in 4 full-term deliveries, with 0 premature births, and 2 abortions or miscarriages, with 3 living children.

This information can be dictated as G6, P4, Ab2 *or* as gravida 6, para 4, abortus 2; transcribe as dictated. G_6P_{4023} is an acceptable style of dictation and transcription as well. If the numbers used in GYN dictation do not "add up," either question it or check the chart.

GPMAL = *g*ravida, *p*ara, *m*ultiple births, *a*bortions, *l*ive births

TPAL = *t*erm infants, *p*remature infants, *a*bortions, *l*iving children

Cardiology Terms

Heart murmurs are written in Arabic numerals.

Example

I heard a grade 3/6 systolic ejection murmur at the left sternal border.

Murmurs go up from grade 1 (barely audible, a low-grade murmur) to grade 6 (the loudest, a high-grade murmur). The virgule, dictated as "over," is placed between the murmur grade and the scale used. The murmur above would equal a grade 3 murmur on a scale of 6.

If a partial unit is dictated, transcribe as follows.

A "grade 2 and a half over 4 murmur" would be transcribed: A grade 2.5 over 4 murmur.

A "grade 4 to 5 over 6 murmur" would be transcribed: A grade 4 to 5 over 6 murmur.

Jr, Sr, II, and III

The use of a comma before and a period after Jr and Sr is optional, but use both or neither. At Hillcrest we use *neither*. No comma is used before the ordinal in a proper name.

Examples

Ronald DiVitori Jr
Dafnis Panagides Sr
Sigmund Klein II
Steve Dittman III

CMTips are compiled by Patricia A. Ireland, CMT, FAAMT; references include the AAMT Book of Style *(2nd ed.),* The Gregg Reference Manual *(9th ed.)* Dorland's Illustrated Medical Dictionary *(29th ed.), and* Stedman's Medical Dictionary *(26th ed.).*

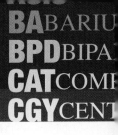

The Student Activities CD-ROM that accompanies the text-workbook contains additional exercises to help you build on the skills required for transcription. The CD-ROM contains various activities such as word building, spelling, image labeling, hangman, and crosswords that allow you to practice and build your medical terminology skills.

The CD-ROM is also designed to assist you in your transcription of the patient cases, reports, and letters described in the text-workbook and contained on the audio transcription exercises. It includes templates for each of the reports used in *Hillcrest Medical Center.* The disk contains a file for each of the following reports: History and Physical, Request for Consultation, Radiology Report, Operative Report, Pathology Report, Discharge Summary, Death Summary, and Autopsy Report. You will also see files for the outpatient reports used in *Quali-Care Clinic,* Hillcrest Medical Center's satellite ambulatory care center. These are the HPIP (history, physical, impression, plan) report, the SOAP (subjective, objective, assessment, plan) report, and correspondence. Tips for formatting your reports are located under "Report Formatting Guidelines" within this section.

Because of the number of files you will be creating as you work through *Hillcrest Medical Center* and *Quali-Care Clinic,* you will need "work" disks on which to save your transcribed reports. We suggest that once you install the program onto your computer's hard drive, you save your reports by cases onto "work" disks. If necessary, refer to your computer user's manual for disk formatting and copying instructions.

After you have transcribed your report to disk, you will want to save the file with an identifiable name. For example, some sample file names could be: H&P-C1 (H&P for "history and physical," C1 for "case 1"), DS-C10 (DS for "discharge summary," C10 for "case 10") and RAD3C10 (RAD for "radiology report," 3 for "radiology report number 3," C10 for "case 10"). Again, refer to your word processing software user's manual if you have questions about saving and naming files.

After keying your medical reports and correspondence, you will want to proofread and spellcheck your reports for accuracy, just as you will need to carefully check your work after you enter the job market.

Report Formatting Guidelines

1. Use two spaces after colons within the body of a report. Do not include spaces after dictator initials in the sign-off block.

2. Double space between all paragraphs.

3. Display all dates on report headings and in the sign-off block as MM/DD/YYYY (*not* M/D/YYYY or M/DD/Y). Dates appearing within the body of a report should be transcribed as dictated (e.g., May 14).

4. Use left justification on reports. (An embedded code has been added to the template disk that will format reports with left justification.)

5. Avoid hyphenation at the end of lines in reports.

6. Use a 1-inch margin on sides, top, and bottom of report pages.

7. Double space between the last line on a page and the "(Continued)" notation.

8. All page breaks should take place between paragraphs or in the middle of a paragraph with at least *two* lines on the bottom of one page and *two* lines at the top of the next page. Avoid "widows" and "orphans" (single lines of text that appear at the bottom or top of a page, separated from the rest of the paragraph).

9. Do not include the signature block alone on a page. Include at least *two* lines of text on the top of the page containing the signature block.

10. Quadruple space (four hard returns) between the ending paragraph of a report and the signature rule (or line).

11. Bring the signature rule back to the left margin. The signature rule for Hillcrest should consist of 25 underscore lines.

12. Do not include extra spaces between the physician's name and the signature rule. The physician's name should be positioned at the left margin to align with the signature rule.

13. Use a double space between the physician's name and the sign-off block at the end of a report.

14. Use a double space between the transcribed date and copy line (if applicable) at the end of a report.

15. Single space all subsequent page headers (report title in all caps, patient name, hospital number, date, and page number). Use a quadruple space to the paragraph below.

16. Use a double space above and below sign-off blocks occurring between two parts of a report.

17. For subheadings containing enumerated text within the body of a report, format the subhead in all caps with a colon.

18. Use all caps and either a colon or a verb for brief introducers within the body of a report (e.g., "HEENT: Normocephalic" used in History and Physical report). Use all caps without a colon for introducers used in a complete sentence (e.g., "SKIN is warm and dry to the touch" used in History and Physical report).

Common Microsoft Word Commands

The chart on this page lists common commands used in Microsoft Word. These commands are displayed to assist you in transcribing medical documents.

Voice Recognition Technology

Voice (or speech) recognition technology is designed to save time, reduce transcription costs, accelerate billing and collection, and offer more flexibility and accuracy to the originator of the dictation.

Some professionals in medical transcription have felt that this technology would *replace* them. However, the transcriptionist will still be needed and will play an important role as medical language specialist and medical/technical editor. The important things for MT students to recognize is that they are studying to enter an important profession, one that is suffering from a lack of well-trained practitioners. Their services will continue to be required, and students are encouraged to think of themselves as medical/technical editors in training.

The future will always hold changes. Voice recognition technology plus medical language specialists will potentially be able to help those in health care by providing accurate patient records in a timely fashion.

Some of the most common prefixes, combining forms, and suffixes used in medical terminology are listed next, with their definitions. Students who have completed a medical terminology course prior to beginning Hillcrest will find this section to be a comprehensive review.

MICROSOFT WORD KEYBOARD COMMANDS			
Action	**Keystrokes**	**Action**	**Keystrokes**
Apply bold	Ctrl+B	Increase font size	Ctrl+Shift+>
Apply italics	Ctrl+I	Increase font size by 1 point	Ctrl+]
Apply underline	Ctrl+U	Indent	Ctrl+M
Cancel	Esc	Justify	Ctrl+J
Center	Ctrl+E	Left align	Ctrl+L
Change case of letters	Shift+F3	Open	Ctrl+O
Change font	Ctrl+Shift+F	Print	Ctrl+P
Change font size	Ctrl+Shift+P	Quit Word	Alt+F4
Close	Ctrl+W	Redo or repeat an action	Ctrl+Y
Copy	Ctrl+C	Reduce hanging indent	Ctrl+Shift+T
Create hanging indent	Ctrl+T	Remove indent from the left	Ctrl+Shift+M
Create new document	Ctrl+N	Remove paragraph formatting	Ctrl+Q
Decrease font size	Ctrl+Shift+<	Right align	Ctrl+R
Decrease font size by 1 point	Ctrl+[	Save	Ctrl+S
Double-space lines	Ctrl+2	Single-space lines	Ctrl+1
Format letters as all capitals	Ctrl+Shift+A	Undo	Ctrl+Z

Understanding Medical Terminology

Medical terminology appears to be complicated until one learns the principles of basic word structure. Medical terminology consists of the following components.

- prefix, word beginning
- suffix, word ending
- root word, the foundation of a word
- combining vowel, a vowel (usually o) connecting a root word to a suffix or a root word to another root word
- combining form, the combination of a root word and a combining vowel

The combining vowel aids in pronunciation.

Principles

1. Generally speaking, begin reading a medical word from the suffix to the root word and/or prefix.

   Example: **hemi/**   **gloss/**   **ectomy**

   half   tongue   removal
   (prefix)   (root)   (suffix)

   Definition: removal of half (one side of) the tongue

2. Drop the combining vowel before a suffix beginning with a vowel.

   Example: **gastr/**   **itis**   **NOT gastr/**   **o/**   **itis**

   stomach   inflammation
   (root)   (suffix)

   Definition: inflammation of the stomach

3. Retain the combining vowel before a suffix beginning with a consonant.

   Example: **gastr/**   **o/**   **megaly**   **NOT gastr/**   **megaly**

   enlargement
   (suffix)

   Definition: enlargement of the stomach

4. Retain the combining vowel between two root words even if the second root word begins with a vowel.

   Example: **electr/**   **o/**   **encephal/**   **o/**   **graphy**

   electricity   brain   process of recording
   (root)   (root)   (suffix)

   Definition: process of recording the electricity of the brain

Prefixes, Pronunciation

Prefixes/Pronunciation	Meaning	Example
A		
a- (ā, ă)	not, without	apnea—not breathing
ab- (ăb)	away from	aberrant—deviating from the normal
ad- (ăd)	to, toward	adhere—to cling together
ambi- (ăm′ bǐ)	on both sides	ambilateral—affecting both sides
an- (ăn)	not, without	anoxia—without oxygen
ante- (ăn′ tē)	before	antefebrile—before the onset of fever
anti- (ăn′ tī, an′ tǐ)	against	antiemetic—an agent that prevents nausea
auto- (aw′ tō)	self	autohypnotic—pertaining to self-induced hypnotism
B		
bi- (bī)	two	biarticular—pertaining to two joints
brady- (brăd′ ē, brād′ ē)	slow	bradycardia—slowness of the heartbeat
C		
cata- (kăt′ ah)	down	cataphoria—a permanent downward turning of the visual axes of the eyes
co- (kō)	with, together	cohesive—uniting together
con- (kŏn)	with, together	confluent (kon′ floo-ŭnt) becoming merged
contra- (kŏn′ trah)	against, opposite	contraceptive—an agent that prevents conception
D		
de- (dē)	lack of	dehydrate—to remove water from
di- (dī)	two, twice	diplopia—double vision
dia- (dī′ ah)	complete, through	dialysis—complete separation
dis- (dĭs)	reversal, separation	disacidify—to remove an acid from
dys- (dĭs)	bad, painful, difficult	dysmenorrhea—painful menstrual flow
E		
ecto- (ĕk′ tō)	out, outside	ectopic—out of normal position
en- (ĕn)	in, within	encephalic—within the skull
endo- (ĕn′ dō)	within	endocrine—pertaining to secretions within
epi- (ĕp′ ǐ)	above, upon	epibulbar—upon the eyeball
eu- (ū)	good, well, easily	eupepsia—good digestion
ex- (ĕks)	out, outside	excision—removal
exo- (ĕk′ sō)	outside, outward	exocardial—situated outside the heart
H		
hemi- (hĕm′ ē)	half	hemiglossitis—inflammation of one half of the tongue
hyper- (hī′ pĕr)	above, excessive	hyperactivity—excessive activity
hypo- (hī′ pō)	deficient, below	hypotension—abnormally low blood pressure

Prefixes/Pronunciation	Meaning	Example
I		
in (ĭn)	not	incurable—not able to be cured
infra- (ĭn′ frah)	below, inferior	infrasternal—below the sternum (breast bone)
inter- (ĭn′ tĕr)	between	intercostal—between the ribs
intra- (ĭn′ trah)	within	intracutaneous—within the skin
M		
macro- (măk′ rō)	large	macrocyte—an abnormally large erythrocyte (red blood cell)
mal- (măl)	bad	malnutrition—any disorder of nutrition
meso- (mĕz′ ō)	middle	mesonasal—situated in the middle of the nose
meta- (mĕt′ ah)	beyond, change	metamorphoses—change of shape
micro- (mī′ krō)	small	microcyst—a very small cyst
N		
neo- (nē′ ō)	new	neonate—a newborn infant
P		
pan- (păn)	all	panhysterectomy—total hysterectomy
para- (păr′ ah)	near, beside	paraesophageal—near the esophagus
per- (pĕr)	through	percutaneous—performed through the skin
peri- (pĕr ē)	around, surrounding	perihepatic—occurring around the liver
poly- (pŏl′ ē)	many	polyneuritis—inflammation of many nerves
post- (pōst)	after, behind	postoperative—after a surgical procedure
pre- (prē)	before, in front of	preprandial—before meals
pro- (prō)	before	prognosis—a forecast as to the probable outcome of a disease
R		
re- (rē)	back, again	reabsorb—to absorb again
retro- (rĕt′ rō)	behind, backward	retronasal—behind the nose
S		
semi- (sĕm′ ē)	one half, partly	semiprone—partly prone (lying face downward)
sub- (sŭb)	under, below	subabdominal—situated below the abdomen
supra- (soo′ prah)	above, over	suprarenal—situated above a kidney
sym- (sĭm)	together, with	sympodia—fusion of the lower extremities
syn- (sĭn)	together, with	syndrome—a set of symptoms that occur together
T		
tachy- (tăk′ ē)	fast, rapid	tachycardia—rapid heartbeat
trans- (trăns)	across, through	transepidermal—occurring through or across the epidermis (top layer of skin)
U		
ultra- (ŭl′ trah)	beyond, excess	ultrastructure—the structure beyond the resolution power of the light microscope

(Continued)

Combining Forms

Combining Form	Meaning	Example
A		
aden/o (ăd′ ĕn-ō)	gland	adenodynia—pain in a gland
angi/o (ăn′ jē-ō)	vessel	angiectomy—surgical excision of a vessel
arteri/o (ăr-tē′ rē-ō)	artery	arterioplasty—surgical repair of an artery
arthr/o (ăr′ thrō)	joint	arthrotomy—surgical incision of a joint
B		
blephar/o (blĕf′ ăr-ō)	eyelid	blepharoplegia—paralysis of an eyelid
brachi/o (brā′ kē-ō)	arm	brachiocephalic—pertaining to the arm and head
bucc/o (bŭk′ ō)	cheek	buccolingual—pertaining to the cheek and tongue
burs/o (bŭr′ sō)	bursa (fluid-filled sac)	bursopathy—any disease of a bursa
C		
carcin/o (kăr′ sĭn-ō)	carcinoma	carcinolysis—destruction of carcinoma cells
cardi/o (kăr′ dēō)	heart	cardiogenic—originating in the heart
cephal/o (sĕf′ ah-lō)	head	cephaledema—edema of the head
cerebr/o (sĕr′ ĕ-brō)	brain, cerebrum	cerebrospinal—pertaining to the brain and spinal cord
cervic/o (sĕr′ vĭ-kō)	neck	cervicoplasty—plastic surgery of the neck
coccyg/o (kŏk′ sĭ-gō)	tailbone, coccyx	coccygodynia—pain in the coccyx
cost/o (kŏs′ tō)	ribs	costoclavicular—pertaining to the ribs and clavicle (collar bone)
crani/o (krā′ nē-ō)	skull	craniopathy—any disease of the skull
cutane/o (kūt-tā′ nē-ō)	skin	subcutaneous—beneath the skin
cyst/o (sĭs′ tō)	urinary bladder	cystogram—an x-ray of the urinary bladder
D		
dactyl/o (dăk′ tĭl-ō)	finger or toe	dactylospasm—spasm of a finger or toe
dent/i (dĕn′ tē)	tooth	dentibuccal—pertaining to the teeth and cheek
dips/o (dĭp′ sō)	thirst	dipsosis—morbid thirst
dors/o (dōr′ sō)	back of the body	dorsolateral—pertaining to the back and side
E		
electr/o (e-lĕk′ trō)	electricity	electrotome—a surgical cutting instrument powered by electricity
encephal/o (ĕn-sĕf′ ah-lō)	brain	encephalomyelitis—inflammation of the brain and spinal cord
enter/o (ĕn′ tĕr-ō)	intestine	enterorrhaphy—repair or suture of the intestine
esophag/o (ĕ-sŏf′ ă-gō)	esophagus	esophagomalacia—softening of the walls of the esophagus
F		
fasci/o (făsh′ ē-ō)	fascia (fibrous tissue)	fasciitis—inflammation of fascia
femor/o (fĕm′ ō-rō)	femur (thigh bone)	femoroiliac—pertaining to the femur and ilium (hip bone)
fibul/o (fĭb′ ū-lō)	fibula (the smaller of the two lower leg bones)	fibulocalcaneal—pertaining to the fibula and calcaneus (heel bone)

Combining Form	Meaning	Example
G		
gastr/o (găs′ trō)	stomach	gastrostenosis—contraction or shrinkage of the stomach
gingiv/o (jĭn′ jĭ-vō)	gums	gingivolabial—pertaining to the gums and lips
gloss/o (glŏs′ ō)	tongue	glossopharyngeal—pertaining to the tongue and pharynx (throat)
gynec/o (gī′ nĕ-kō)	woman, female	gynecology—that branch of medicine that treats diseases of the female genital tract
H		
hemat/o (hēm′ ah-tō)	blood	hematuria—blood in the urine
hepat/o (hĕp′ ah-tō)	liver	hepatologist—a specialist in the study of the liver
hist/o (hĭs′ tō)	tissue	histolysis—destruction of tissue
hypn/o (hĭp′ nō)	sleep	hypnogenic—inducing sleep
hyster/o (hĭs′ tĕr-ō)	uterus, womb	hysterosalpingectomy—excision of the uterus and uterine (fallopian) tubes
I		
idi/o (ĭd′ ē-ō)	individual, self	idiopathic—self-originated condition of unknown causation
ile/o (ĭl′ ē-ō)	ileum (portion of the small intestine)	ileocecal—pertaining to the ileum and cecum
ili/o (ĭl′ ē-ō)	ilium (expansive superior portion of the hip bone)	iliocostal—pertaining to the ilium and ribs
J		
jejun/o (jĕ-joo′ nō)	jejunum (portion of the small intestine)	jejunectomy—excision of the jejunum
K		
kerat/o (kĕr′ ah-tō)	cornea	keratomycosis—fungal infection of the cornea
kinesi/o (kĭ-nē′ sē-ō)	movement	kinesiotherapy—treatment of disease by movements or exercise
L		
labi/o (lā′ bē-ō)	lip	labiolingual—pertaining to the lips and tongue
laryng/o (lah-rĭng′ ō)	larynx (voice box)	laryngoparalysis—paralysis of the larynx
later/o (lăt′ ĕr-ō)	side	lateroversion—a turning to one side
lip/o (lĭp′ ō)	fat, lipid	lipiduria—lipids in the urine
lith/o (lĭth′ ō)	stone, calculus	lithogenous—producing or causing the formation of calculi
M		
mamm/o (măm′ ō)	breast	mammoplasty—plastic reconstruction of the breast
mast/o (măs′ tō)	breast	mastography—the making of an x-ray of the breast
my/o (mī′ ō)	muscle	myobradia—slow, sluggish reaction of muscle to electric stimulation
myel/o (mī′ ĕ-lō)	spinal cord, bone marrow	myelopoiesis—formation of bone marrow

Combining Form	Meaning	Example
N		
nas/o (nā′ zō)	nose	nasopalatine—pertaining to the nose and palate (roof of the mouth)
nephr/o (nĕf′ rō)	kidney	nephrorrhagia—hemorrhage from a kidney
neur/o (nū′ rō)	nerve	neuroallergy—allergy in nervous tissue
noct/i (nŏk′ tē)	night	nocturia—excessive urination at night
O		
onc/o (ŏng′ kō)	mass, tumor	oncogenesis—the production or causation of tumors
oo/o (ō′ ō-ō)	egg, ovum	oocyte—an immature egg
oophor/o (ō-ŏf′ ō-rō)	ovary	oophorohysterectomy—excision of the ovaries and uterus
ophthalm/o (ŏf-thăl′ mō)	eye	ophthalmodynia—pain in the eye
orchi/o (ŏr′ kē-ō)	testis, testicle	orchitis—inflammation of the testicle
or/o (ō′ rō)	mouth	oral—pertaining to the mouth
oste/o (ŏs′ tē-ō)	bone	osteodystrophy—abnormal, defective bone formation
ot/o (ō′ tō)	ear	otorrhea—a discharge from the ear
ox/o (ŏk′ sō)	oxygen	anoxia—absence of oxygen
P		
path/o (păth′ ō)	disease	pathoanatomic—pertaining to the anatomy of diseased tissue
poster/o (pŏs′ tĕr-ō)	back (of the body)	posterolateral—behind and to one side
pseud/o (sū′ dō)	false	pseudocyesis—false pregnancy
psych/o (sī′ kō)	mind	psychogenesis—mental development
py/o (pī′ ō)	pus	pyosalpinx—pus in the uterine tube
R		
radi/o (rā′ dē-ō)	rays, x-rays	radioimmunity—diminished sensitivity to radiation
ren/o (rē′ nō)	kidney	renal—pertaining to the kidney
retin/o (rĕt′ ĭ-nō)	retina	retinomalacia—softening of the retina
rhin/o (rī′ nō)	nose	rhinotomy—incision of the nose
roentgen/o (rĕnt′ gĕn-ō)	x-rays	roentgenotherapy—treatment with roentgen rays
S		
sacr/o (sā′ krō)	sacrum	sacrodynia—pain in the sacral region
salping/o (săl-pĭng′ gō)	uterine tubes	salpingo-oophorectomy—excision of a uterine tube and an ovary
secti/o (sĕk′ shē-ō)	to cut	section—a cut surface
sphygm/o (sfĭg′ mō)	pulse	sphygmometer—an instrument for measuring the pulse
stomat/o (stō′ mah-tō)	mouth	stomatomycosis—fungal disease of the mouth

Combining Form	Meaning	Example
T		
thorac/o (thō′ rah-kō)	chest	thoracoscopy—examination of the pleural cavity with an endoscope
tibi/o (tĭb′ ē-ō)	tibia, shin bone (the larger of the two lower leg bones)	tibialgia—painful shin bone
top/o (tŏp′ ō)	place, position, location	ectopic—located away from normal position
tox/o (tŏk′ sō)	poison	toxicity—the quality of being poisonous
trache/o (trā′ kē-ō)	trachea (windpipe)	tracheolaryngotomy—incision of the larynx (voice box) and trachea
U		
ur/o (ū′ rō)	urine, urinary tract	urolith—a calculus (stone) in the urine
uter/o (ū′ tĕr-ō)	uterus	uteroplacental—pertaining to the placenta and uterus
V		
vagin/o (văj′ ĭ-nō)	vagina	vaginovesical—pertaining to the vagina and urinary bladder
vas/o (văs′ ō)	vessel, duct	vasomotion—change in the caliber of a (blood) vessel
ven/o (vē′ nō)	vein	veno-occlusive—pertaining to obstruction of the veins
viscer/o (vĭs′ ĕr-ō)	internal organs	viscerad—toward the viscera
X		
xanth/o (zăn′ thō)	yellow	xanthemia—presence of yellow coloring matter in the blood
xer/o (zēr′ rō)	dry	xerosis—abnormal dryness
Z		
zyg/o (zī′ gō)	yoked, joined	zygal—shaped like a yoke

Suffixes

Suffix	Meaning	Example
A		
-ac (ăk)	pertaining to	cardiac—pertaining to the heart
-al (ăl)	pertaining to	postnatal—pertaining to after a birth
-algia (ăl′ jē-ah)	pain	otalgia—pain in the ear
-asthenia (ăs-thē′ nē-ah)	lack of strength	myasthenia—lack of muscular strength
C		
-cele (sēl)	hernia	cystocele—hernial protrusion of the urinary bladder through the vaginal wall
-centesis (sĕn-tē′ sĭs)	surgical puncture to remove fluid	amniocentesis—surgical puncture to remove fluid from the amnion
-cidal (sī′ dăl)	killing	bactericidal—destructive to bacteria
-clysis (klī′ sĭs)	irrigation, washing	enteroclysis—irrigation of the bowel
-coccus (kōk′ ŭs)	bacterial cell	staphylococcus—microorganism that causes localized suppurative infections
-cyte (sīt)	cell	leukocyte—white blood cell
D		
-desis (dē′ sĭs)	binding	arthrodesis—surgical fixation of a joint
E		
-ectasis (ĕk′ tah-sĭs)	stretching, dilation	angiectasis—lengthening of a blood vessel
-ectomy (ĕk′ tō-mē)	removal	appendectomy—removal of the vermiform appendix
-emesis (ĕm′ ĕ-sĭs)	vomiting	hyperemesis—excessive vomiting
-emia (ē′ mē-ah)	blood condition	septicemia—blood poisoning
G		
-genesis (jĕn′ ĕ-sĭs)	producing, originating	pathogenesis—the development of disease or a morbid condition
-gram (grăm)	record	myelogram—an x-ray of the spinal cord
-graph (grăf)	instrument for recording	gastrograph—an instrument for recording the motions of the stomach
-graphy (grăf′ ē)	process of recording	myelography—process of recording an x-ray of the spinal cord
I		
-ia (ē′ ah)	condition, process	dyspepsia—condition of bad digestion
-ic (ĭk)	pertaining to	thoracic—pertaining to the chest
-ist (ĭst)	specialist	nephrologist—a specialist in the study of the kidney
-itis (ī′ tĭs)	inflammation	osteitis—inflammation of a bone
L		
-logy (lō′ jē)	study of	ophthalmology—study of the eye
-lysis (lī′ sĭs)	separation, destruction	splenoylysis—destruction of splenic tissue

Suffix	Meaning	Example
M		
-malacia (mah-lā′ shē-ăh)	softening	osteomalacia—softening of bone
-megaly (mĕg′ ah-lē)	enlargement	acromegaly—enlargement of extremities
O		
-odynia (ō-dĭn′ ē-ah)	pain	gastrodynia—pain in the stomach
-ole (ōl)	little, small	arteriole—a minute arterial branch
-oma (ō′ mah)	tumor	carcinoma—a malignant new growth
-opia (ō′ pē-ah)	vision	amblyopia—dimming of vision
-orrhaphy (ŏr′ ah-fē)	suture	herniorrhaphy—suture of a hernia
-orrhea (ō′ rē-ah)	flow, discharge	menorrhea—discharge of the menses
-osis (ō′ sĭs)	abnormal condition	arthropyosis—abnormal condition of pus in a joint cavity
-osmia (ŏz′ mē-ah)	smell	anosmia—absence of the sense of smell
-ostomy (ŏs′tō-mē)	new opening	colostomy—surgical creation of a new opening in the colon
P		
-pepsia (pĕp′ sē-ah)	digestion	dyspepsia—bad digestion
-phagia (fā′ jē-ah)	eating, swallowing	polyphagia—excessive eating
-phobia (fō′ bē-ah)	fear	hydrophobia—fear of water
-plasia (plā′ zē-ah)	formation, development	chondroplasia—the formation of cartilage
-plasty (plăs′ tē)	surgical repair	rhinoplasty—surgical repair of the nose
-plegia (plē′ jē-ah)	paralysis	hemiplegia—paralysis of one side of the body
-pnea (nē′ ah)	breathing	dyspnea—difficult breathing
-ptosis (tō′ sĭs)	drooping, prolapse	blepharoptosis—drooping of the eyelid
-ptysis (tĭ′ sĭs)	spitting	hemoptysis—spitting blood
S		
-sclerosis (sklē-rō′ sĭs)	hardening	arteriosclerosis—hardening of the arteries
-scope (skōp)	instrument for visual examination	cystoscope—an instrument for visual examination of the urinary bladder
-stasis (stā′ sĭs)	control, stop	hemostasis—stopping the flow of blood
-stenosis (stĕn-ō′ sĭs)	narrowing, stricture	angiostenosis—narrowing of a vessel
T		
-therapy (thĕr′ ah-pē)	treatment	thermotherapy—therapeutic use of heat
-tocia (tō′ sē-ah)	labor, birth	dystocia—abnormal labor
-tome (tōm)	instrument to cut	osteotome—an instrument to cut bone
-tomy (tō′ mē)	incision	tracheotomy—incision of the trachea
-trophy (trō′ fē)	nourishment, development	hypertrophy—excessive development
U		
-ule (ūl)	little, small	venule—a small vein
-uria (ū′ rē-ah)	urination, urine	pyuria—pus in the urine

SECTION 4
Case Studies

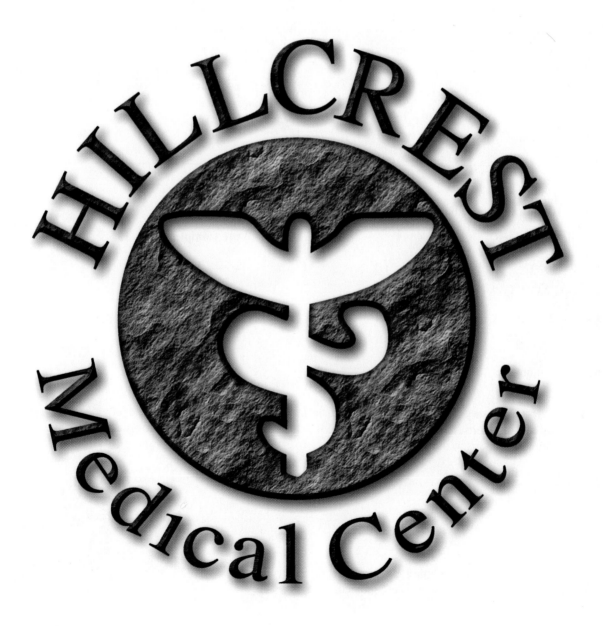

Patient Name
Brenda C. Seggerman

Address
701 Dadeland Blvd.
Miami, FL 33133-5017

Situation
Brenda Seggerman's vaginal spotting and abdominal pain had increased during the night until she was in an emergent situation, and her husband called an ambulance. Once in the Hillcrest emergency room, the patient was assessed. A pregnancy test was found to be positive. Further testing by radiology revealed an ectopic pregnancy. Her gynecologist was called, and the patient was prepared for immediate surgery. Tissues removed at surgery were sent to pathology for examination and final diagnosis. After three days Mrs. Seggerman was discharged to office followup in improved condition.

Review Figures CS1-1A and B, The Female Anatomy; Figure CS1-2, Continuous Suturing Technique; and Figure CS1-3, Sites of Ectopic Pregnancy on pages 67–68.

Student Name _____

Patient: Brenda C. Seggerman

Sequence of Reports	Date Completed	Grade
Emergency Services Admission Report	_____	_____
Diagnostic Imaging Report	_____	_____
Operative Report	_____	_____
Pathology Report	_____	_____
Discharge Summary	_____	_____

NOTE: Study the glossary for Case 1. Enter the date each report is completed in the space provided. When you have transcribed all reports, tear this sheet out, staple it to the front of the reports (in the order listed above); give the completed reports to the instructor.

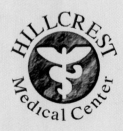

Glossary for Case 1

adhesions (ăd-hē′zhens)—fibrous bands or structures by which body parts abnormally adhere, as in wound healing

adnexa (sing. and pl.) (ăd-nĕk′sah)—appendages or adjunct parts (primarily used in the plural form)

adnexal mass (ăd-nĕk′sĕl măs)—an abnormality in the adnexa

approximate (v) (ah-prok′sĭ-māt″)—to bring close together or into apposition

arthralgia (ar-thrăl′jē-ah)—pain in a joint

bimanual (bī-′man-ye-wel)—performed using both hands

blood type O blood type O has neither A nor B antigens

chromic suture (krō′mĭk soo′cher)—absorbable catgut suture material

Claforan (klăh′for-an)—antibiotic against gram-negative bacteria, trade name

crown-rump length—the length between the top of the head to the buttocks or gluteal region

cul-de-sac [Fr.] (kŭl-dŭh-săk′)—a blind pouch

Demerol (dĕm′er-ol)—trade name for meperidine hydrochloride, a preoperative drug to sedate and relieve pain

distal (dĭs′tal)—farther from any point of reference

ectopic pregnancy (ĕk-tŏp′ĭk)—a pregnancy in which the fertilized ovum becomes implanted on tissue outside of the uterine cavity

edema (ĕ-dē′mah)—abnormal accumulation of fluid in the intercellular tissue spaces of the body, resulting in swelling

embedment (ĕm-bĕd′ment)—a tissue specimen that is fixated in a firm medium to keep it intact during sectioning of the tissue

endovaginal (ĕn″dō-văj′ĭ-nal)—within the vagina

EtOH—ethyl alcohol; ethanol; grain alcohol

exploratory laparotomy (lăp″ah-rŏt′ō-mē)—surgical abdominal resection to gain access to the peritoneal cavity

fallopian tube (făl-lō′pē-ăn)—also called oviduct or uterine tube; transports the ovum from the ovary to the uterus

fascia (făsh′ē-ah)—supportive layer of thin connective tissue within the muscles and/or organs of the body

figure-of-eight stitches—sutures in which the thread follows the contours of the figure eight

fundus (fŭn′dŭs)—the bottom or base of anything; the part of an organ opposite the opening into that organ

general endotracheal tube (ĕn″dō-trā′kē-ăl)—referring to the tube inserted within the trachea through which to administer general anesthesia

gravida 2 [L.], para 1 [L.], abortus 1 [L.] (grăv′ĭ-dah) (păr′ah) (ah-bor′tŭs)—two pregnancies; one live birth; one abortion or miscarriage

gravida 3, para 1-0-2-1—three pregnancies; one live birth, no premature births, two abortions or miscarriages, and one living child

GYN—abbreviation for gynecology

Heaney clamp (hā′nē)—medical tool used to grasp and manipulate tissue

HEENT—head, eyes, ears, nose, throat

hematemesis (hēm″ah-tĕm′ĕ-sĭs)—the vomiting of blood

hematochezia (hĕm-ăh″tō-kē″zē-ah)—the passage of bloody stools

hematocrit (Hct) (hē-măt′ō-krĭt)—the volume percentage of erythrocytes in whole blood

hematuria (hĕm″ah-tū′rē-ah)—blood in the urine

hemoglobin (Hgb) (hē′mō-glō″bĭn)—carries oxygen from the lungs to the tissues and carbon dioxide from the tissues to the lungs

hemoperitoneum (hē″mō-per″ĭ-tō-nē′um)—an effusion of blood in the peritoneal cavity

hemostasis (hē″mō-stā′sĭs)—the arrest of bleeding by surgical means

ICD code: 633.1—International Classification of Diseases; a standard list of identifying codes used in statistics, billing, etc. (This code refers to an ectopic pregnancy.)

informed consent—a patient gives written permission for surgery, clinical treatment, and/or to release his or her records to a third party after a thorough discussion of the issues with the physician involved

lactated Ringer's (solution)—a fluid and electrolyte replenisher given to a patient by intravenous infusion

lyse (v) (līse)—to cut or separate, as at surgery

lysis of adhesions (lī′sĭs)—disintegration or destruction of adhesions (a surgical procedure)

melena (mĕl′ĕ-nă)—the passage of black stools

mesosalpinx (mēz″ō-săl′pĭnks)—layers that enclose a uterine tube, which are composed of the broad ligament of the uterus and are located above the mesovarium

mucopurulent (mū″kō-pū′roo-lĕnt)—containing both mucus and pus

No. 1 (suture)—referring to the size of suture materials (see "Suture Sizing" in Section 3 on page 50)

normal saline—a 0.9% solution of sodium chloride

oriented x3—neurologic terminology meaning that a patient is aware of place, person, and time

packing laps—cloths used to pack off the tissues and aid in hemostasis during surgery, also called laparotomy pack

palpable (păl′pah-b′l)—perceptible by touch

pelvic (pĕl′vĭk)—referring to the pelvis, the basinlike structure formed by the hips, and all it contains

pelvic ultrasound—an imaging study of the pelvic area in which the deep structures of the pelvis are scanned by way of ultrasonic waves for diagnostic purposes

peritoneum (per″ĭ-tō-nē′um)—the serous membrane lining the abdominal walls and investing the viscera

Pfannenstiel incision (făn′ĕn-stēēl)—abdominal incision curved in a downward "smile" at the bikini line; named for Dr. Hermann Johann Pfannenstiel, a German gynecologist

Phenergan (fĕn′ĕr-găn)—medicinal sedative and antinauseant, trade name

pilonidal cyst (pī″lō-nī′dal)—a cyst containing a nidus or tuft of hairs, usually found at the base of the spine

positive cardiac activity—medical term for "the heart is beating" and all that the statement implies

proximal—nearest; closer to any point of reference

pseudodecidual sign (soo″dō-dē-sĭd′ū-al)—a false response of endometrium in the absence of pregnancy

pseudogestational sac (soo″dō-jĕs-tā′shĕn-al)—false pregnancy; the gestational sac surrounds the embryo, but in a false pregnancy there is a "pseudo" or false gestational sac

retractor—instrument used to hold wound edges and/or tissues apart during surgery

Rh negative—describes people *with no* Rh antigen in their blood

Rh positive—describes people *with* the Rh antigen in their blood

RhoGAM (rō′găm)—trade name for a preparation of $Rh_0(D)$ immune globulin, required in an Rh-negative mother

ruptured tubal pregnancy—a pregnancy in a fallopian tube that has burst through the walls of the tube

salpingectomy (săl″pĭn-jĕk′tō-mē)—surgical removal of a uterine tube

serosal abrasion (sē-rō′săl)—the wearing away of the serous membrane

speculum (spĕk′ū-lŭm)—instrument used to spread open a passage or a cavity for ease in its examination

staple gun—an instrument by which one accomplishes the process of fastening a surgical opening with staples

subcutaneous (sŭb″kū-tā′nē-ŭs)—beneath the skin

transabdominal (trans-ăb-dŏm′ĭ-nal)—across or through the abdominal wall

transvaginal ultrasound (trăns-văj′ĭ-nal)—an imaging study utilizing sound waves performed through the vagina (radiologic procedure)

tubo-ovarian (too″bō-ō-vā′rē-ŭn)—pertaining to a uterine tube and ovary

tubo-uterine (too″bō-ū′ter-ĭn)—pertaining to a uterine tube and the uterus

urinalysis (ū″rĭ-năl′ĭ-sĭs)—physical, chemical, or microscopic analysis or examination of urine

uterine adnexa (ū′ter-ĭn ăd-nĕk′sah)—the uterine appendages: the ovaries, uterine tubes, and ligaments of the uterus

Vicryl (vī′krĭl)—trade name for polyglactin 910, an absorbable suture made of multifilament braided material

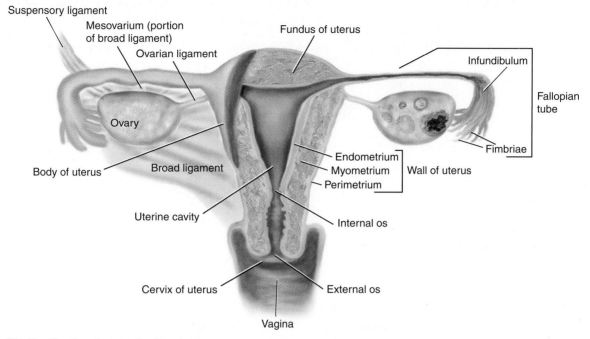

Figure CS1-1A **The female reproductive system.**

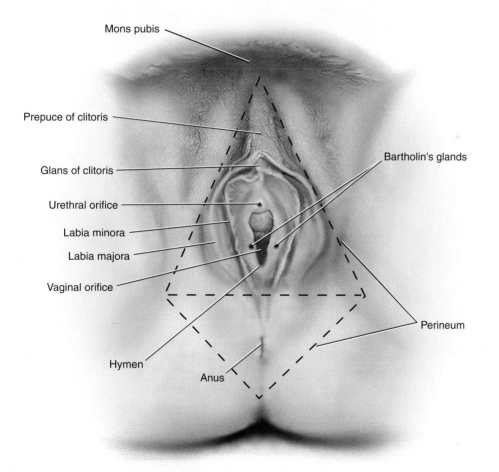

Figure CS1-1B **The female anatomy external genitalia.**

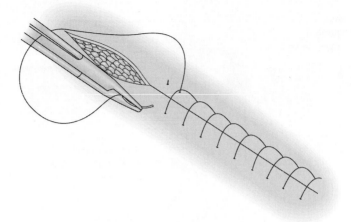

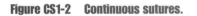

Figure CS1-2   Continuous sutures.

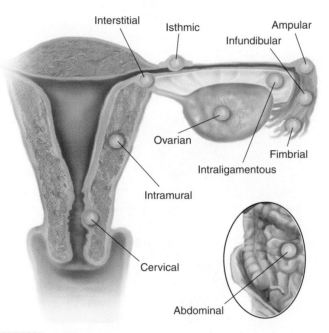

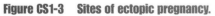

Figure CS1-3   Sites of ectopic pregnancy.

BA BARIU
BPD BIPA
CAT COM
CGY CEN

Patient Name
Emma Parker

Address
938 Shore Road
Ocean View, FL 33140-4989

Situation
This elderly woman fell and injured her hip. She was taken to Hillcrest emergency room where the ER physician ordered an x-ray. Her family physician was called, who requested an orthopedic surgeon to consult. Surgical intervention was decided upon, and the patient was taken to the operating room. Radiology kept a close check on this patient throughout her hospital stay. She developed some cardiac problems postoperatively, and a cardiologist was requested to consult. Social workers at Hillcrest helped to get the patient placed in a nursing home at discharge, where she would be followed by her family physician, orthopedist, and cardiologist.

Review Figure CS2-1, Anterior and Posterior Views of the Adult Human Skeleton; Figure CS2-2, Male and Female Pelvises; and Figure CS2-3, Right Hipbone on pages 71–72.

Student Name _____

Patient: Emma Parker

Sequence of Reports	Date Completed	Grade
History and Physical Examination	_____	_____
Radiology Report	_____	_____
Operative Report	_____	_____
Discharge Summary	_____	_____

NOTE: Study the glossary for Case 2. Enter the date each report is completed in the space provided. When you have transcribed all reports, tear this sheet out, staple it to the front of Hillcrest reports (in the order listed above); give completed reports to the instructor.

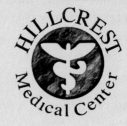

Glossary for Case 2

abduct (ăb-dŭkt′)—to draw or pull a part of the body away from the median axis

Accu-Chek (ăk′ū-chĕk)—trade name for a blood sugar monitor (equipment)

ADA—American Diabetes Association

Ancef (ăn′sĕf)—trade name for cefazolin, an antibiotic

anicteric (ăn″ĭk-tĕr′ĭk)—without icterus (jaundice; yellow appearance)

anteversion (ăn″tē-vĕr′zhŭn)—forward displacement of an organ

antibiotic (ăn″tĭ-bī-ŏt′ĭk)—chemical substance produced by a variety of microorganisms; used to destroy or inhibit the growth of bacteria and/or other microorganisms

AP—refers to *anteroposterior* direction, from front to back

appendectomy—surgical removal of the vermiform appendix

AST—*as*partate *t*ransaminase (an enzyme) newer name for and sometimes dictated in place of SGOT

bipolar (bī-pō′lăr)—having two poles, ends, or extremes

buccal (bŭk′ăl)—pertaining to the inside of the cheek

C-arm images—results of portable x-ray unit used in the operating room; the C-shaped unit is made to surround the part being studied

chronic—persisting over a long period of time

click—a brief sharp sound (heart sound)

copious (kō′pē-ŭs)—yielding something abundantly

cortical (kor′tĭ-kăl)—pertaining to a cortex (outer layer of an organ or other body structure)

CPK *c*reatine *p*hospho*k*inase (a lab test done on blood)

DePuy sliding screw (du′pwee)—orthopedic device used in femoral fracture repair

dissect (dĭ-sĕkt′)—to cut apart or separate

dyspnea (dĭsp′nē-ah)—difficult or labored breathing

electrocautery (ē-lĕk″trō-kaw′tĕr-ē)—the application of an electric current to destroy or cut through tissue

endotracheal (ĕn″dō-trā′kē-ăl)—within or through the trachea

EOMI—*e*xtra*o*cular *m*uscles (or movements) *i*ntact

external rotation—movement of an external appendage about its axis, e.g., moving either the leg or the arm in a circle

fascia lata (făsh′ē-ah lah′tah)—the external layer of fascia (supportive layer of thin connective tissue) of the thigh

femoral (fĕm′ŏr-ăl)—pertaining to the femur (thigh)

flex—to bend

fluoroscopy (floo″ŏr-ŏs′kō-pē)—examination using a fluoroscope (an instrument used for examining deep structures by means of roentgen rays)

funduscope (fŭn′dŭs-skōp)—an instrument for examining the fundus (bottom or base) of the eye

gallop (găl′ŏp)—an abnormal rhythm of the heart

H&H—*h*emoglobin and *h*ematocrit (blood tests, part of a complete blood count)

Hemovac drain (hē′mō-văc)—a closed suction drainage unit to evacuate blood and serum postoperatively, trade name

infarct (ĭn′fărkt)—necrosis (death) of a tissue due to local ischemia (obstruction of blood)

intact (ĭn-tăkt′)—remaining uninjured or unimpaired

intercostal (ĭn″tĕr-kŏs′tăl)—situated between the ribs

interrupted sutures—sutures (surgical stitches) that are placed separately and tied separately

intertrochanteric fracture (ĭn″tĕr-trō″kăn-tĕr′ĭk)—a break within the trochanter (bones of the neck of the femur or thigh)

ischemia (ĭs-kē′mē-ah)—obstruction of blood to a body part due to a pathologic condition

IVPB—*i*ntra*v*enous *p*iggy*b*ack (to infuse fluids, medicines, etc., into the body through an IV already established)

lateralis [L.] (lăt″ĕr-ā′lĭs)—pertaining to one side; a point of reference farther from the midplane of the body

LDH—*l*actic *de*hydrogenase (a lab test done on blood)

Lowman turkey-claw clamp (lō′măn)—orthopedic equipment used during surgery

MI—*m*yocardial *i*nfarction (heart attack)

Micronase (mī′krō-nās)—trade name for glyburide; used in the management of type 2 diabetes mellitus

myocardial (mī″ō-kăr′dē-ăl)—pertaining to the myocardium (muscular tissue of the heart)

Nitro-Dur (nī′trō dŭr)—trade name for nitroglycerin; used in treating angina pectoris and other cardiac problems

nondiaphoretic (nŏn-dī″ah-fō-rĕt′ĭk)—no profuse perspiration

normocephalic (nōr″mō-sĕ-făl′ĭk)—pertaining to a normal-sized head

OR—*o*perating *r*oom

organomegaly (ŏr″gah-nō-mĕg′ă-lē)—enlargement of one or more of the viscera (internal organs)

ORIF—*o*pen *r*eduction, *i*nternal *f*ixation (of a fracture)

PERRLA—*p*upils *e*qual, *r*ound, and *r*eactive to *l*ight and *a*ccommodation

plane—an imaginary flat surface used for description or depiction; anatomists identify three planes of the body, i.e., frontal, sagittal, and transverse

PMI—*p*oint of *m*aximal *i*mpulse (cardiac term)

prominence (prŏm′ĭ-nĕns)—a protrusion or projection

prosthesis (prŏs-thē′sĭs)—an artificial replacement for a missing body part, such as eye, an arm, or a leg

reamer (rē′mĕr)—an instrument used in orthopedic surgery to enlarge an artificial orifice or passage in bone

renal insufficiency—inability of the kidneys to remove nitrogenous wastes adequately

rhonchus (rŏng′kŭs)—a rattling sound in the lower respiratory tract heard on auscultation (pl. rhonchi)

rub (pericardial rub) (pĕr″ĭ-kăr′dē-ăl rŭb)—a scraping or grating noise heard with the heartbeat

sclera (sklē′rah)—the sturdy white outer layer of the eyeball (pl. sclerae)

SGOT—*s*erum *g*lutamic-*o*xaloacetic *t*ransaminase (a lab test done on blood); see AST

ST-T waves—describes heart function on an electrocardiogram (EKG); there are P, Q, R, S, T, and U waves

TM—*t*ympanic *m*embrane (in the ear); eardrum

type and cross x2—medical jargon referring to the fact that the patient's blood type needs to be determined in the laboratory, then crossmatched against two units of blood. This blood will be held for the patient's needs during surgery. If not needed, it will be released for crossmatch against another patient's blood.

UA—*u*rin*a*lysis (or urine analysis)

vastus lateralis (văs′tŭs lăt″ĕr-ā′lĭs)—a large muscle overlying the hip joint and anterolateral thigh

Wygesic (wī-jē′zĭk)—trade name for a narcotic pain medication (acetaminophen and propoxyphene)

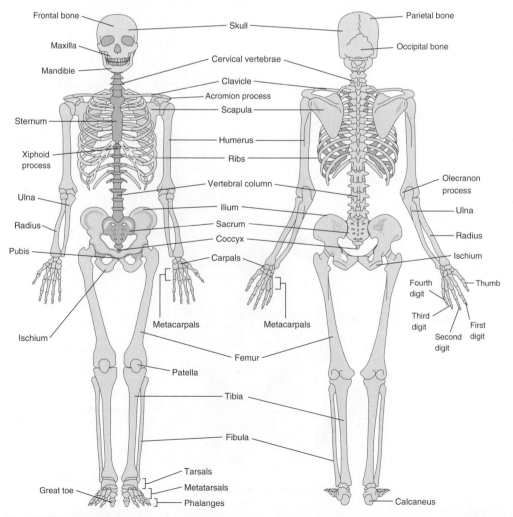

Figure CS2-1   The adult human skeleton.

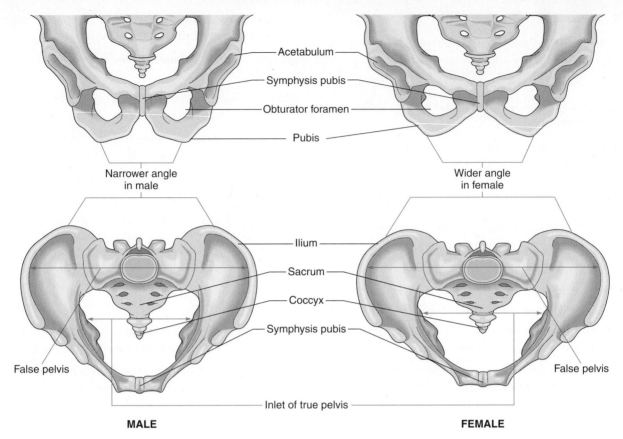

Figure CS2-2   The male and female pelvic structure.

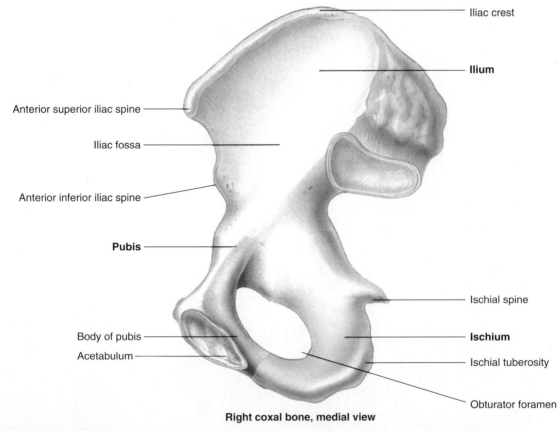

Right coxal bone, medial view

Figure CS2-3   The hipbone.

ASIAN
BABARIU
BPDBIPA
CATCOM
CGYCEN

Patient Name
Putul Barua

Address
3506 NW 56th Court
North Miami Beach, FL 33160-5938

Situation
Putul Barua, a middle-aged man from Bangladesh, presented to Hillcrest Medical Center with signs and symptoms of a possible myocardial infarction. He was admitted to Cardiac Care and evaluated by both cardiology and pulmonology. Workup showed the patient to have hemoptysis with a history of tuberculosis. Further testing included bronchoscopy, CT scan of chest, chest x-ray, CT scan of brain, and an open lung biopsy. The patient developed renal failure, which was managed by nephrology. Mr. Barua did not improve; he was pronounced dead on hospital day eight. Permission for autopsy was denied.

Review Figure CS3-1, The Cardiopulmonary System; Figure CS3-2, Acute Myocardial Infarction; and Figure CS3-3, General or Systemic Circulation.

Student Name _____

Patient: Putul Barua

Sequence of Reports	Date Completed	Grade
History and Physical Examination	_____	_____
Operative Report	_____	_____
Diagnostic Imaging Report 1	_____	_____
Diagnostic Imaging Report 2	_____	_____
Diagnostic Imaging Report 3	_____	_____
Death Summary	_____	_____

NOTE: Study the glossary for Case 3. Enter the date each report is completed in the space provided. When you have transcribed all reports, tear this sheet out, staple it to the front of the reports (in the order listed above); give completed reports to the instructor.

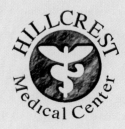

Glossary for Case 3

acute hepatic failure (ah-kūt′ hĕ-păt′ĭk)—the sudden onset of liver failure

alveolitis (ăl″vē-ō-lī′tĭs)—inflammation of alveoli (air sacs in the lung)

amphoric (am-for′ĭk)—a hollow sound resulting from percussion over a lung cavity

asystolic (ā″sĭs-tol′ĭk)—absence of a heartbeat

atrial fibrillation (ā′trē-al fi″brĭ-lā′shun)—rapid, irregular contractions of the atria (upper chambers of the heart)

atrial flutter (ā′trē-al flŭt′er)—rapid contractions of the atria, more regular than fibrillation

axial sections (ăk′sē-ăl)—referring to the parts of the brain examined by CT scan, which is done in sections throughout the center of the brain

axillary (ăk′sĭ-ler″ē)—pertaining to the armpit

basal ganglia calcifications (bā′săl găng′lē-ah)—deposits of calcium in basal ganglia (groups of nerve cells in the brain)

bilateral (bī-lăt′er-al)—occurring on both sides

bleb (blĕb)—an abnormal air-filled sac in emphysematous lung tissue

bronchoscopy (brŏng-kŏs′kō-pē)—examination of the bronchi through a bronchoscope (a surgical procedure)

brushings (brŭsh′ĭngs)—to obtain cell samples using a brush; this material can be sent for histologic or cytologic evaluation

carina (kah-rī′nah)—a ridgelike structure where the trachea divides into the left and right main stem bronchi

cavitary lesions (kăv′ĭ-tar″ē lē′zhŭns)—abnormal tissue areas containing cavities

cerebral edema (sĕ-rē′brăl ĕ-dē′mah)—excessive accumulation of fluid in the brain substance that causes swelling

Code Blue—medical jargon meaning a patient's heartbeat and/or respirations have ceased, calling for immediate resuscitation procedures (CPR)

congestion—swelling of blood vessels due to engorgement with blood

cords—referring to the vocal cords

cortical atrophy (kor′tĭ-kal ăt′rō-fē)—death of cells in the cerebral cortex (part of the brain)

Coumadin (koo′mah-dĭn)—trade name for warfarin sodium, an anticoagulant drug

CT—abbreviation for computed tomography

CT scan—a procedure in which x-ray images are analyzed and combined by a computer to yield views representing thin slices of the part examined

dialysis catheter (dī-ăl′ĭ-sĭs kăth′ĕ-ter)—tubular instrument inserted into a major vein in order to filter the blood of impurities; done in patients whose kidneys have less than normal function

dilatation (dĭl″ah-tā′shŭn)—the condition of being stretched (dilated) beyond normal dimensions

echocardiogram (ĕk″ō-kăr′dē-ō-grăm)—an image produced by recording an echo obtained from beams of ultrasonic waves directed through the chest wall and bouncing back from the heart (cardio); it depicts the structures of the heart

effusion (ĕ-fū′zhŭn)—the escape of fluid into a body part or tissue

ejection fraction—the proportion of the volume of blood in the ventricles at the end of diastole that is ejected during systole

EKG leads—conductors connected to an electrocardiograph (EKG) machine

embolectomy (ĕm″bō-lĕk′tō-mē)—surgical removal of a blood clot (embolus) from a blood vessel

endobronchial (ĕn″dō-brŏng′kē-ăl)—within the bronchi

epiglottis (ĕp″ĭ-glŏt′ĭs)—the lidlike cartilaginous structure that folds back over the opening of the windpipe during swallowing, which prevents food from entering the lungs

ET tube—abbreviation for endotracheal tube, a tube inserted into the trachea (windpipe) to assist in ventilating the patient

etiology (ē″tē-ŏl′o-jē)—cause or origin of a disease or disorder

fungemia (fŭn-jē′mē-ah)—the presence of a fungal growth in the blood stream

gastrostomy tube (găs-trŏs′tō-mē)—tube inserted through a surgical opening into the stomach, through which nutrition and medication are supplied to the patient

glottis (glŏt′ĭs)—the opening between the vocal cords and the larynx

Hemoccult (hē′mō-kŭlt)—trade name for a test to discover occult (hidden) blood in the stool

hemodialysis (hē″mō-dī-ăl′ĭ-sĭs)—the removal of waste substances from the blood by means of a hemodialyzer

hemoptysis (hē-mŏp′tĭ-sĭs)—the expectoration or spitting up of blood or blood-stained sputum

hepatosplenomegaly (hĕ-pah″tō-splē″-nō-mĕg′ah-lē)—enlargement of the liver and spleen

high-flow oxygen—oxygen administered to a patient via the highest setting on the oxygen machine (as opposed to low-flow oxygen, which is at a lower setting)

hilar (hī′lĕr)—pertaining to the depression, notch, or opening where the vessels and nerves enter an organ

HPI—abbreviation for history of present illness

hydrocephalus (hī″drō-sĕf′ah-lŭs)—an increase in the volume of cerebrospinal fluid in the ventricles of the cerebrum

hypokinesia (hī″pō-kĭ-nē′zē-ah)—abnormally decreased motor function or activity

hypoxemic (hī″pŏk-sē′mĭk)—pertaining to deficient oxygenation of the blood

idiopathic pulmonary fibrosis (ĭd″ē-ō-păth′ĭk pŭl′mō-ner-ē fī-brō′sĭs)—hardening of the pulmonary (lung) structures of either unknown or spontaneous origin

infiltrate (ĭn-fĭl′trāt)—(v) to penetrate small openings of a tissue or substance; (n) when present on chest x-ray it indicates pneumonia

INR—international normalized ratio (see laboratory discussion on page 000)

intraoperatively (ĭn″trah-ŏp′ĕr-ă-tĭv-lē)—during an operative procedure (surgery)

intravenous (ĭn″trah-vē-′nŭs)—within or through a vein

intravenous contrast—material inserted into a vein that allows differences in tissues to be delineated; used in radiology and cardiology procedures

intubated (ĭn′tū-bāt-ĕd)—the condition of having a tube inserted into a body canal or hollow organ

intubation (ĭn″tū-bā′shŭn)—the insertion of a tube into a body canal or hollow organ

Klebsiella pneumoniae (klĕb″sē-ăl′ah nū mō-nē-ī)—one etiologic agent of acute bacterial pneumonia (microbiology genus and species name)

lesion (lē′zhŭn)—a traumatic break in tissue or a pathologic loss of function of a part of the body

low-flow oxygen—oxygen administered to a patient via the lowest setting on the oxygen machine (as opposed to high-flow oxygen, which is at a higher setting)

lymphadenopathy (lĭm-făd″ĕ-nŏp′ah-thē)—disease of the lymph nodes

malaise (mal-āz′)—a vague feeling of bodily discomfort

mechanical ventilation—ventilation (breathing) supported or provided by a machine

mediastinal (mē″dē-ah-stī′năl)—pertaining to the membranous partition separating the lungs or the two pleural sacs

MVA—abbreviation for motor vehicle accident

myocardial infarction (mī″ō-kăr′dē-ăl ĭn-fărk′shŭn)—gross necrosis of the myocardium due to lack of blood supply to the area (heart attack)

nephrologist (nĕ-frŏl′ō-jĭst)—a specialist in the study of the kidney

open-lung biopsy—taking a small sample of apparently diseased tissue in surgery while the lungs are exposed (as opposed to a brush biopsy or a procedure with the lungs not exposed)

palpitation(s) (păl″pī-tā′shŭns)—rapid or irregular heartbeat(s), primarily used in the plural form

parenchymal (pah-rĕng′kĭ-mal)—pertaining to the essential elements of an organ, i.e., the functional elements of an organ

pleural (ploo′răl)—pertaining to the serous membrane that covers the lungs and lining of the thoracic cavity

prothrombin time (prō-thrŏm′bĭn)—a test for coagulation factors of the blood (see laboratory discussion on pages 198–199)

pseudocords (soo″dō-kords)—false cords (long, rounded structures)

pulmonary (pŭl′mō-ner″ē)—pertaining to the lungs

pulmonary vascular congestion—engorgement of pulmonary vessels occurring in cardiac disease, infections, and certain bodily injuries

rhonchus (pl. rhonchi) (rong′kŭs) (rong′kī)—a continuous dry rattling sound (heard on auscultation) in the throat or bronchial tube due to some type of obstruction

S₁, S₂, S₃, S₄ or S1, S2, S3, S4—first, second, third, and fourth heart sounds; may be heard while listening to the heart via stethoscope; S1 and S2 are normal sounds, S3 and S4 are not normally heard

septicemia (sĕp″tĭ-sē′mē-ah)—toxins in the blood, also called blood poisoning

sputum (spū′tŭm)—material coughed up from the lower respiratory tract

subarachnoid hemorrhages (sŭb″ah-răk′nŏid)—hemorrhage (bursting forth of blood) at or between the arachnoid and pia mater of the brain

supraventricular cardiac arrhythmias (soo″prah-vĕn-trĭk′ū-lar kăr′dē-ak ah-rĭth′mē-ahs)—irregularity in the rhythm of the heart starting from a focus above the ventricles

Swan-Ganz catheter (swăn-gănts kăth'ě-ter)—a catheter with a balloon at the tip for measuring pulmonary arterial pressures, trade name

thorax (thō'răks)—chest

thrombosis (thrŏm-bō'sĭs)—formation or presence of a thrombus or blood clot

trachea (trā'kē-ah)—windpipe

tracheostomy (trā''kē-ŏs'tō-mē)—surgical opening into the trachea

tuberculosis (too-ber'kū-lō'sĭs)—an infectious disease of the lung

ventricles (věn'trĭ-k'ls)—lower chambers of the heart

Versed (věr-sěd')—trade name for a nonbarbiturate drug given intravenously (either before or during surgery) to produce sedation and amnesia

WNL—abbreviation for within normal limits

Xylocaine (zī'lō-kān)—trade name for lidocaine, a topical anesthetic drug

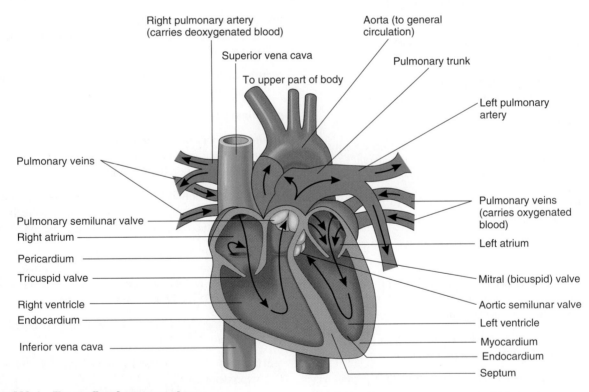

Figure CS3-1   The cardiopulmonary system.

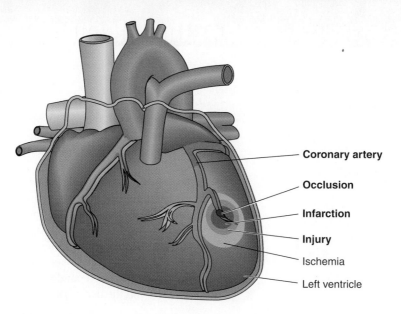

Figure CS3-2   Myocardial infarction.

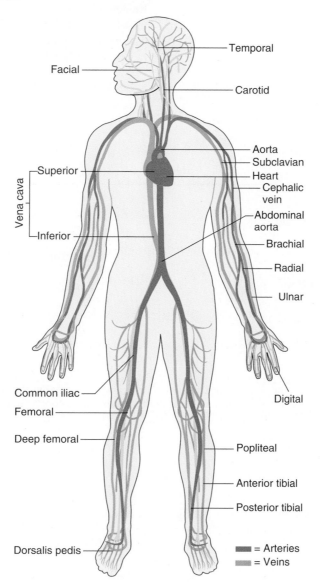

Figure CS3-3   Systemic circulation.

ANTE
ARIUM
BIPAR
COMP
CENTI

Case 4: The Integumentary System

Patient Name
Gloria Ramos

Address
5900 SE 22nd Avenue
Miami Beach, FL 33156-5937

Situation
Gloria Ramos, a middle-aged woman with multiple medical problems, developed painful ulcerations of her mouth and lips, making eating and drinking difficult. She sought medical treatment at her internist's office, and he admitted her to Hillcrest Medical Center. Ms. Ramos had a routine chest x-ray on admission, and she was referred to dermatology services in consultation. The dermatologist and internist agreed on a treatment plan for the patient, and after a few days marked improvement was noted in her condition. She was discharged in improved condition to be followed by the internist and the dermatologist as needed.

Review Figure CS4-1, Anatomy of the skin; Figure CS4-2, Comparison of normal bone to bone with osteoporosis; and Figure CS4-3, The anatomy of the mouth on pages 80–81.

Student Name _____

Patient: Gloria Ramos

Sequence of Reports	Date Completed	Grade
History and Physical Examination	_____	____
Radiology Report	_____	____
Request for Consultation	_____	____
Discharge Summary	_____	____

NOTE: Study the glossary for Case 4. Enter the date each report is completed in the space provided. When you have transcribed all reports, tear this sheet out, staple it to the front of the reports (in the order listed above); give completed reports to the instructor.

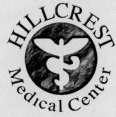

Glossary for Case 4

albeit (ăl-bē'ĭt)—even though

albumin (ăl-bū'mĭn)—a necessary protein substance produced in the liver; levels are reduced in malnutrition and in hepatic and renal diseases

arthritis (ăr-thrī'tĭs)—inflammation of the joints

azathioprine (ā'zah-thī'ō-prēn)—generic drug used in treating rheumatoid arthritis and other autoimmune diseases

Azulfidine (ā-zŭl'fĭ-dēn)—trade name for sulfasalazine, an antibacterial agent

chlorambucil (klō-răm'bū-sĭl)—generic drug used in chemotherapy, an antineoplastic agent

compression fracture—any break or rupture of bone due to compression, e.g., the bones in the spinal column

corticosteroids (kŏr''tĭ-kō-stē'roids)—a group of steroids (or lipids) used clinically in immune suppression, in hormonal replacement, etc.

cyclophosphamide (sī''klō-fŏs'fah-mīd)—generic drug used in chemotherapy, an antineoplastic agent

debilitating—causing weakness or lack of strength

dehydration (dē''hī-drā'shŭn)—condition resulting from either excessive loss or inadequate intake of body water

dermatology (dĕr''mah-tŏl'ō-jē)—the study of the skin

diffuse (dĭ-fūs')—(adj) widely distributed, not concentrated; (v) to pass through or disperse through tissue or body structure

Disalcid (dī-săl'sĭd)—trade name for a nonsteroidal anti-inflammatory drug used to treat minor pain, fever, and arthritis

distally (dĭs'tăl-lē)—in a remote direction; opposite of proximal or near

Dolobid (dō'lō-bĭd)—trade name for diflunisal; used to treat mild to moderate pain

dysphagia (dĭs-fā'jē-ah)—difficulty swallowing

ecchymosis (ĕk''ĭ-mō'sĭs)—a small spot on the skin or mucous membrane forming a nonelevated, blue or purplish patch; a bruise (pl. ecchymoses)

enteritis (ĕn''tĕr-ī'tĭs)—inflammation of the intestine, particularly the small intestine

erosion (ē-rō'zhŭn)—destruction of the surface of the epidermis (skin), which heals without scar tissue

erythema (ĕr''ĭ-thē'mah)—redness of the skin produced by abnormal accumulation of blood

erythema multiforme (mŭl'tĭ-fŏrm''āy)—a symptom complex including multiple skin lesions of varying degrees of severity

exophthalmos (ĕk''sŏf-thăl'mōs)—abnormal protrusion of the eyeball

exudate (ĕks'ū-dāt)—any fluid that has escaped from blood vessels and been deposited in tissues, usually due to an injury or inflammation

fissuring (fĭsh'ūr-ĭng)—splitting, normal or otherwise; can include painful ulcerations

flare—area of redness of the skin

folic acid (fō'lĭk ăs'ĭd)—a B complex vitamin, the lack of which can result in severe anemia and birth defects

gingiva (jĭn'jĭ-vah)—the pale pink tissues of the oral mucosa, otherwise known as the gums

HCTZ—abbreviation for *h*ydrochloro*t*hiazide, a generic diuretic medication used to treat edema and hypertension

hydroxychloroquine (hī-drŏk''sē-klō'rō-kwĭn)—generic drug used to treat rheumatoid arthritis

hyperpigmentation (hī''pĕr-pĭg''mĕn-tā'shŭn)—abnormally increased coloration

hyporeflexia (hī'pō-rē-flĕk'sē-ah)—decreased reflexes

IV hydration—receiving fluids *i*ntra*v*enously

injection (n)—the condition of being congested or overloaded with blood

intravenous (ĭn''trah-vē'nŭs)—within or through a vein

kyphosis (kī-fō'sĭs)—abnormally increased curvature of the thoracic spine; humpback

leucovorin (loo''kō-vō'rĭn)—generic drug used to treat both anemia and malignancies

Lidex gel (lī'dĕks jĕl)—trade name for topically applied gel; an anti-inflammatory agent

liver enzymes (lĭv'ĕr ĕn'zīms)—those protein molecules that induce necessary chemical reactions in the liver; a group of laboratory tests on blood or serum that give the values of these proteins

macular (măk'ū-lăr)—pertaining to the presence of a macule; a nonelevated, discolored spot on the skin

methotrexate—generic chemotherapy drug used also in immunosuppressive disorders

nephrocalcinosis (nĕf''rō-kăl''sĭ-nō'sĭs)—diffusely scattered calcifications in the kidneys leading to renal insufficiency

NSAID—abbreviation for *n*onsteroidal *a*nti-*i*nflammatory *d*rug

osteoporosis (ŏs″tē-ō-pō-rō-́sĭs)—reduction in the amount of bone mass leading to pathologic fractures

palate (păl′ăt)—roof of the mouth

penicillamine (pĕn″ĭ-sĭl′ah-mēn)—generic drug, a product of penicillin; used to treat rheumatoid arthritis

perimalleolar (pĕr″ĭ-măl-ē′ō-lăr)—around the bony protuberances on either side of the ankle

pitting edema—when too much fluid is in the tissues (edema), a finger pressing on the skin leaves pitting indentations or areas of pitting in the skin

p.o. [L.] (pĕr ŏs)—*per os* (by mouth)

posterior pharynx (făr′ĭnks)—the back of the throat

prednisone (prĕd′nĭ-sōn)—generic anti-inflammatory drug

Premarin (prēm′ah-rĭn)—trade name for preparations of estrogen, the female hormone

quiescent—at rest; inactive

regimen (rĕj′ĭ-mĕn)—a strictly regulated plan of therapy, diet, exercise, or other activity designed to achieve a certain goal

rheumatoid arthritis (roo′mah-toid ăr-thrī′tĭs)—chronic systemic, painful joint disease that can result in deformities

serum cholesterol (sē′rŭm kō-lĕs′tĕr-ŏl)—the level of cholesterol (a complex organic compound synthesized in the liver and other tissues) found in the serum; high levels of cholesterol can clog arteries and can form gallstones

stasis edema (stā′sĭs ĕ-dē′mah)—stagnation of the flow of blood or fluids resulting in swelling

Stevens-Johnson syndrome—a severe, sometimes fatal multisystemic form of erythema multiforme

stomatitis (stō-mah-tī′tĭs)—inflammation of the oral mucosa, the mucous membrane of the mouth

t.i.d. [L.] *ter in die* (three times a day)

topically—referring to a surface area; applying a substance to a certain surface area of the skin

total protein—a laboratory test to determine the level of all proteins in the serum

vertebral bodies (vĕr′tĕ-brăl) (vĕr-tē′brăl)—any of the 33 bones of the spinal canal

volume depletion—dehydrated state

Westergren sedimentation rate—standard laboratory test to determine the erythrocyte sedimentation rate (ESR) using a tube and a method designed by Alf Westergren, a Swedish physician born in 1891

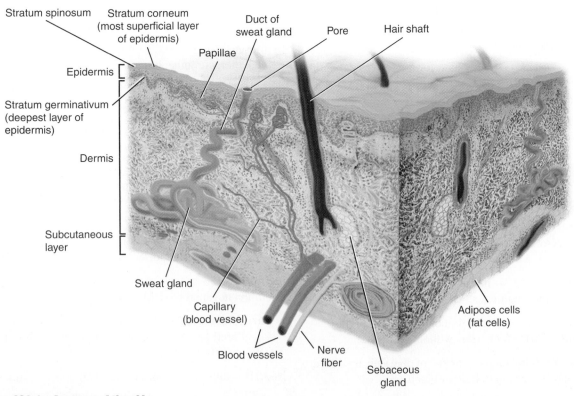

Figure CS4-1   Anatomy of the skin.

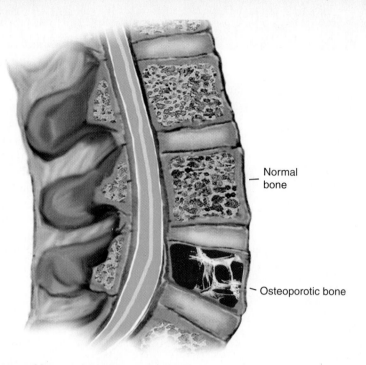

Figure CS4-2   Comparison of normal bone to bone with osteoporosis.

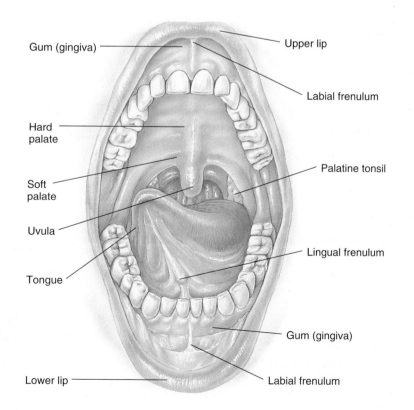

Figure CS4-3   The anatomy of the mouth.

Patient Name
Carlos Lopez

Address
509 Red Road
Miami, FL 33114-0229

Situation
Carlos Lopez is an elderly patient who has suffered with difficulty emptying his urinary bladder. He went to his family physician who referred him to a urologist, a surgeon specializing in the treatment of the urinary tract and the male genitalia. The patient was taken to surgery, and the tissues removed were sent to a pathologist for both macroscopic and microscopic examination and diagnosis. The patient was subsequently discharged from the hospital by his family physician, to be followed as an outpatient by both the family physician and the urologist.

Review Figure CS5-1, The Urinary System; and Figure CS5-2, Structures of the Kidney on page 84.

Student Name _____

Patient: Carlos Lopez

Sequence of Reports	Date Completed	Grade
History and Physical Examination	_____	_____
Operative Report	_____	_____
Pathology Report	_____	_____
Discharge Summary	_____	_____

NOTE: Study the glossary for Case 5. Enter the date each report is completed in the space provided. When you have transcribed all reports, tear this sheet out, staple it to the front of the reports (in the order listed above); give completed reports to the instructor.

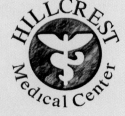

Glossary for Case 5

atrophy (ăt′rō-fē)—a wasting away; a reduction in the size of cell, tissue, organ, or other body part due to a variety of factors such as malnutrition and/or ischemia

autonomic (aw″tō-nŏm′ĭk)—self-controlling, self-governing; functionally independent

Bactrim DS (băk′trĭm)—trade name for a combination antibiotic and sulfonamide anti-infective used for urinary tract, respiratory tract, and ear infections

bruit [Fr.] (brwē) (brōōt)—a sound or murmur heard on auscultation, especially an abnormal one; primarily used in the plural, bruits

BUN—abbreviation for *b*lood *u*rea *n*itrogen (a laboratory test done on blood)

carotid (kah-rŏt′ĭd)—the main artery on either side of the neck that supplies blood to the head and neck

CBC—abbreviation for *c*omplete *b*lood *c*ount

cholecystectomy (kō″lē-sĭs-tĕk′tō-mē)—surgical removal of the gallbladder

corpora amylacea [L.] (kŏr′pō-rah ăm″ĭ-lā′sē-ah)—small hyaline masses of degenerate cells found in the prostate (sing. corpus amylaceum)

creatinine (krē-ăt′ĭ-nĭn)—a waste product of protein metabolism excreted in the urine; a blood test to check kidney function

cystourethroscope (sĭs″tō-ū-rē′thrō-skōp)—an instrument for examining the urinary bladder and posterior urethra

cystourethroscopy (sĭs″tō-ū″rē-thrŏs′kō-pē)—process of visually examining the urinary bladder and posterior urethra

diverticulum (dī″vĕr-tĭk′ū-lŭm)—an abnormal, circumscribed pouch or sac in the intestinal wall (pl. diverticula)

dysuria (dĭs-ū′rē-ah)—painful or difficult urination

efflux (ĕf′lŭks)—a flowing out or emanating

electrocardiogram (EKG) (ē-lĕk″trō-kăr′dē-ō-grăm″)—a graphic tracing of the electrical changes in heart muscle (sometimes abbreviated ECG)

Foley catheter (fō′lē kăth′ĕ-tĕr)—a catheter placed in the bladder and retained by a balloon for the purpose of draining urine from the bladder, trade name

French scale—a scale used for indicating the size of catheters and other tubular instruments, based on a measurement of each unit being approximately equivalent to 0.33 mm in diameter; i.e., 1 mm = #3 French

gastrointestinal (GI) (găs″trō-ĭn-tĕs′tĭ-năl)—pertaining to the stomach and intestine

granuloma (sing.) (grăn″ū-lō′mah)—a tumorlike mass or nodule consisting of granulation tissue (pl. granulomata)

granulomatous (grăn″ū-lōm′ah-tŭs)—composed of granulomata

hyperplasia (hī″pĕr-plā′zē-ah)—an abnormal increase in the number of cells in a tissue or organ

hypotension (hī″pō-tĕn′shŭn)—abnormally low blood pressure

Hytrin (hī′trĭn)—trade name for terazosin, an antihypertensive drug

induration (ĭn′dū-rā′shŭn)—the quality of tissue or an organ being hard; the process of hardening

indwell—to dwell in; reside within

lithiasis (lĭ-thī′ah-sĭs)—the formation of calculi or mineral concretions (solidified masses) within the body

lithotomy (lĭ-thŏt′ō-mē)—incision of a duct or organ, often the urinary bladder, for removal of calculi (stones)

optic fundi (ŏp′tĭk fŭn′dī)—pertaining to the back of the interior of the eyes

orifice (ŏr′ĭ-fĭs)—the opening of any cavity in the body

orthostatic (ŏr″thō-stăt′ĭk)—pertaining to or caused by an upright position

prostate (prŏs′tāt)—a gland in the male that surrounds the neck of the urinary bladder and the urethra

prothrombin (prō-thrŏm′bĭn)—a factor in the blood plasma that combines with calcium to form thrombin during blood clotting

PTT—*p*artial *t*hromboplastin *t*ime; one laboratory test to determine how fast the blood clots

rale [Fr.] (rahl)—an abnormal respiratory sound heard on auscultation, indicating some pathologic condition; primarily used in the plural form; rales

renal (rē′năl)—pertaining to the kidney

resect (rē-sĕkt′)—to surgically remove part of an organ or tissue

resectoscope (rē-sĕk′tō-skōp)—an endoscopic instrument used for transurethral removal or biopsy of lesions of the bladder, prostate, or urethra

sphincter (sfĭngk′tĕr)—a ring-shaped muscle that can open or close a natural orifice by expanding or contracting

splenomegaly (splē″nō-měg′ah-lē)—enlargement of the spleen

stroma (strō′ mah)—the supporting tissue of an organ, as distinguished from its functional element

trabeculate (trah-běk′ū-lāt)—marked with cross bars

trabeculation (trah-běk″ū-lā′shŭn)—the formation of trabeculae (strands of connective tissue) in a part

transurethral resection (TUR) (trăns″ū-rē′thrăl rē-sěk′shŭn)—a surgical procedure to relieve urinary ob-

struction by reaming out the enlarged part of the gland that is encroaching on the urethra and blocking the outflow of urine

van Buren sounds—surgical instruments used to dilate a structure or to detect a foreign body, named after Dr. William van Buren

void (v)—to eliminate as waste matter

wheeze—an abnormal whistling sound made during respiration

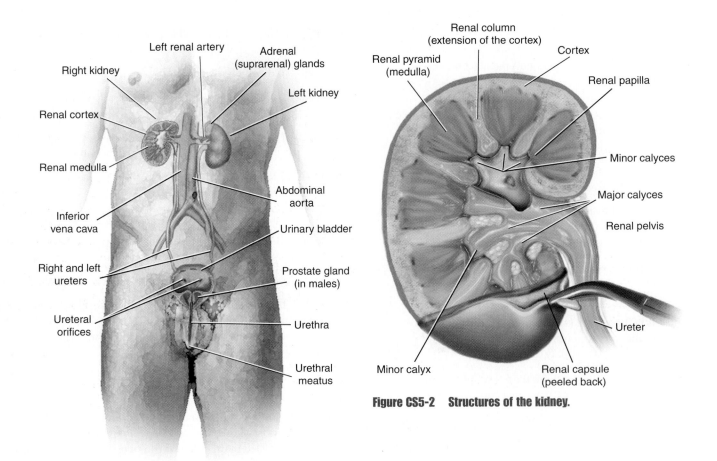

Figure CS5-1   Structures of the urinary system.

Figure CS5-2   Structures of the kidney.

Patient Name
Lydia Cruz

Address
7334 Kendall Avenue
Miami, FL 33156-5948

Situation
After suffering with long-term pain in both her low back and right leg and receiving no benefit from chiropractic manipulation, Ms. Cruz sought advice and treatment from a neurosurgeon. She was admitted to Hillcrest for radiology testing, which revealed her to have a herniated disk. She was taken to surgery where the herniated disk was removed and the tissue sent to pathology for examination and diagnosis. After an uneventful, afebrile hospital course, the patient was discharged in improved condition with her pain resolved.

Review Figure CS6-1, Spinal Column; Figures CS6-2A, Typical Vertebra and B, Herniated Disk; Figure CS6-3, Joint Movements; Figure CS6-4, Spinal Nerves; and Figure CS6-5, Cranial Nerves on pages 88–92.

Student Name _____

Patient: Lydia Cruz

Sequence of Reports	Date Completed	Grade
History and Physical Examination	_____	_____
Radiology Report 1	_____	_____
Radiology Report 2	_____	_____
Operative Report	_____	_____
Pathology Report	_____	_____
Discharge Summary	_____	_____

NOTE: Study the glossary for Case 6. Enter the date each report is completed in the space provided. When you have transcribed all reports, tear this sheet out, staple it to the front of the reports (in the order listed above); give completed reports to the instructor.

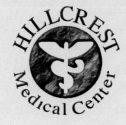

Glossary for Case 6

aggregating—crowding or clustering together

ambulating (ăm″bū-lā′tĭng)—walking

arthropathy (ăr-thrŏp′ah-thē)—any joint disease

blunted—to make less sharp; dull

cesarean (sē-sār′ē-ăn)—referring to cesarean section, an incision through the abdominal and uterine walls for delivery of a fetus

chiropractor (kī′rō-prăk′tŏr)—a practitioner of chiropractic, a conservative science of applied neurophysiology; e.g., chiropractic theory is that irritation of the nervous system is the cause of disease

Cloward saddle (klow′ĕrd)—surgical equipment in which a patient is placed for back fusion, trade name

contrast medium—a substance that is introduced into or around a structure and, because of the difference in absorption of x-rays by both the contrast medium and the surrounding tissues, allows radiographic visualization of the structure (pl. contrast media)

contused (kŏn-tūzd′)—bruised

convex (kŏn′vĕks)—having a surface that is rounded and somewhat elevated

curette (kū-rĕt′)—spoon-shaped surgical instrument for removing tissue from a cavity wall or other bodily surface

Darvocet (dăr′vō-sĕt)—trade name for drug used to treat mild to moderate pain

denies x3—this phrase, as used in the Social History, refers to the fact that the patient denies alcohol, tobacco, and illicit drug use

discrete—made up of separate and distinct parts or defined by lesions that do not become unified

diskectomy—(dĭs-kĕk′tō-mē)—excision of an intervertebral disk (is sometimes spelled discectomy)

epinephrine (ĕp″ĭ-nĕf′rĭn)—generic drug used as a vasoconstrictor, cardiac stimulant, and bronchodilator; also called adrenaline

exacerbate (ĕg-zăs′ĕr-bāt″)—to increase in severity

facet (făc-et′)—a small, smooth surface on a bone or other hard anatomic body

Flexeril (flĕks′ĕr-ĭl)—trade name for drug used to treat muscle spasm

focal degeneration—main area or center of deterioration

formalin (fŏr′mah-lĭn)—a powerful disinfectant gas, used in water as a fluid to preserve tissue removed at surgery for pathologic evaluation; same as formaldehyde

Gelfoam sponge—trade name for absorbable gelatin sponge; sterile, they are used in surgery to stop the flow of blood

gutter—low area, trough, or groove

herniated (hĕr′nē-āt″ĕd)—protruding like a hernia; enclosed in a hernia

i.e. [L.] *id est* (that is)

intermittent—periodically stopping and starting again at separated intervals

intervertebral (ĭn″tĕr-vĕr′tĕ-brăl) (ĭn″tĕr-vĕr tē′brăl)—located between two adjoining vertebrae

Kantrex (kăn′trĕks)—trade name for an antibiotic

2+ knee and ankle jerks—this phrase refers to the sudden reflex or involuntary movements made when the doctor uses a rubber hammer to tap the knees and ankles; part of the neurologic exam; in this case they are graded as 2+, which means average or normal

L1-2—*l*umbar spine, between first and second vertebrae (the disk space)

L2-3—*l*umbar spine, between second and third vertebrae (the disk space)

L3-4—*l*umbar spine, between third and fourth vertebrae (the disk space)

L4-5—*l*umbar spine, between fourth and fifth vertebrae (the disk space)

L5-S1—*l*umbar spine, fifth vertebra, and *s*acral spine, first vertebra (where the lumbar and sacral spines join)

lamina (lăm′ĭ-nah)—a thin, flat plate or supportive layer, part of the structure of a vertebra

laminectomy (lăm″ĭ-nĕk′tō-mē)—excision of the posterior arch of a vertebra

lateral recess syndrome—a small hollow or indentation on the side of the fourth ventricle; by way of this recess, part of the fourth ventricle protrudes into the subarachnoid space

ligamentum flavum [L.] (lĭg″ah-mĕn′tŭm flāv′ŭm)—band of yellow elastic tissue that assists in maintaining or regaining the erect position between two adjoining vertebrae

light touch—when the doctor lightly strokes a part of the body, such as the extremities, to determine the patient's ability to feel; used in evaluation of the central nervous system

lumbosacral (lŭm″bō-sā′krăl)—pertaining to the lumbar region of the spine (between the thorax and the pelvis) and the sacrum

Marcaine (măr-kān′)—trade name for the local, injectable anesthetic agent bupivacaine

myelogram (mī′ĕ-lō-grăm)—an x-ray of the spinal cord obtained after injection of dye into the spinal canal

Norflex (nŏr′flĕks)—trade name for a drug used to treat muscle spasms

PAR—abbreviation for *post*anesthesia *r*ecovery, where patients are sent immediately after surgery (the recovery room)

pinprick—when the doctor actually pricks a patient's skin with a sharp point to determine the level of feeling; part of the evaluation of the central nervous system

pleura (ploor′ah)—a serous membrane lining the thoracic or pleural cavity

prone (prōn)—lying face downward

radicular (rah-dĭk′ū-lăr)—of or pertaining to a radical, which would be the cause or root of a morbid process, such as radical surgery

retraction—to draw back; the condition of being drawn back, such as tissue during a surgical procedure

rongeur [Fr.] (raw-zhŭr′)—a surgical instrument used for cutting tough tissue, such as bone

S1 root—*s*acral spine, first vertebra, at the lowest part

sacroiliac (sā″krō-ĭl′ē-ăk)—the sacral and iliac spines—where they join and their associated ligaments

scaphoid (skăf′oid)—literally shaped like a boat, a scaphoid bone

scoliosis (skō″lē-ō′sĭs)—a sideways deviation in the normally straight vertical line of the spine (S-shaped spine)

spurring—projecting bodies (outgrowths) from a bone or muscle

straight-leg raising—the doctor observes the patient's ability to raise the legs; part of the evaluation of the central nervous system

subarachnoid space (sŭb″ah-răk′noid spās)—space under the arachnoid membrane, between it and the pia mater

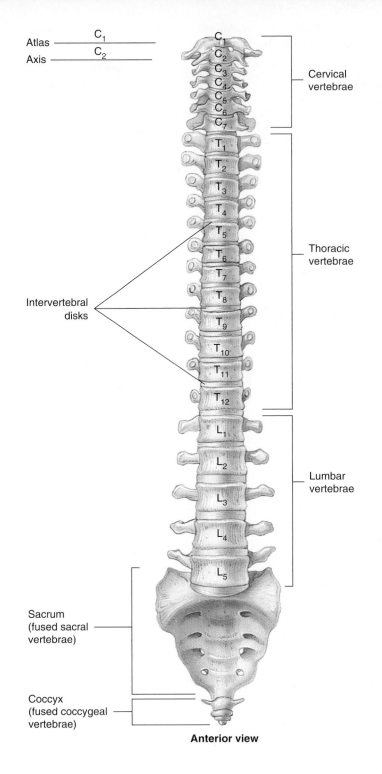

Atlas ——— C₁
Axis ——— C₂

C₁
C₂
C₃
C₄
C₅
C₆
C₇

Cervical vertebrae

T₁
T₂
T₃
T₄
T₅
T₆
T₇
T₈
T₉
T₁₀
T₁₁
T₁₂

Thoracic vertebrae

Intervertebral disks

L₁
L₂
L₃
L₄
L₅

Lumbar vertebrae

Sacrum (fused sacral vertebrae)

Coccyx (fused coccygeal vertebrae)

Anterior view

Figure CS6-1   The spine.

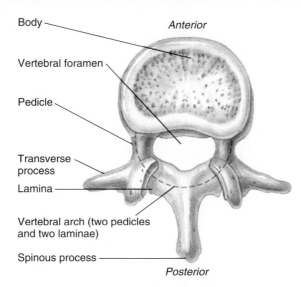

Body

Anterior

Vertebral foramen

Pedicle

Transverse
process

Lamina

Vertebral arch (two pedicles
and two laminae)

Spinous process

Posterior

Superior view

Figure CS6-2A   Typical vertebra.

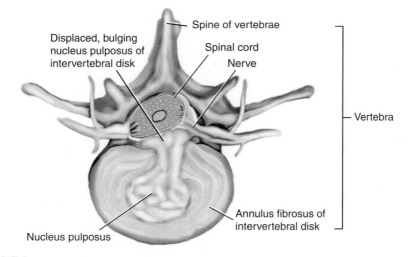

Spine of vertebrae

Displaced, bulging
nucleus pulposus of
intervertebral disk

Spinal cord

Nerve

Vertebra

Annulus fibrosus of
intervertebral disk

Nucleus pulposus

Figure CS6-2B   Herniated disk.

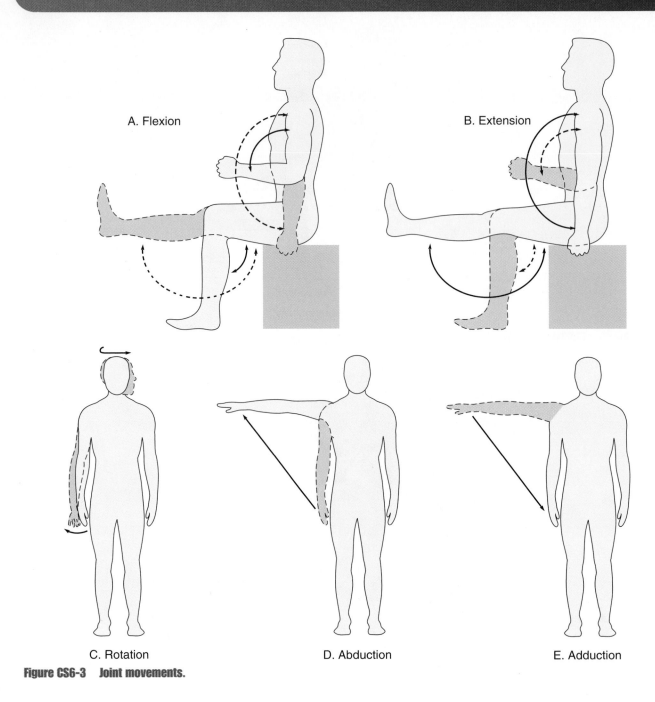

A. Flexion

B. Extension

C. Rotation

D. Abduction

E. Adduction

Figure CS6-3   Joint movements.

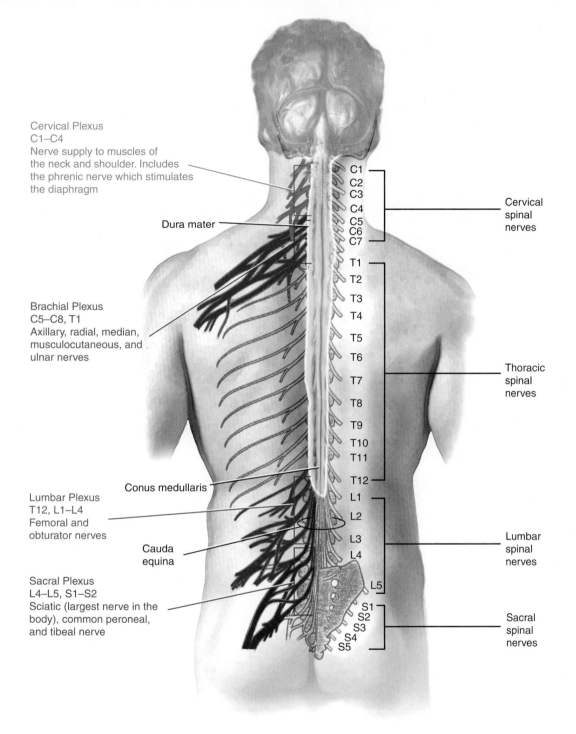

Cervical Plexus
C1–C4
Nerve supply to muscles of
the neck and shoulder. Includes
the phrenic nerve which stimulates
the diaphragm

Dura mater

Brachial Plexus
C5–C8, T1
Axillary, radial, median,
musculocutaneous, and
ulnar nerves

Conus medullaris

Lumbar Plexus
T12, L1–L4
Femoral and
obturator nerves

Cauda
equina

Sacral Plexus
L4–L5, S1–S2
Sciatic (largest nerve in the
body), common peroneal,
and tibeal nerve

C1
C2
C3
C4
C5
C6
C7

Cervical
spinal
nerves

T1
T2
T3
T4
T5
T6
T7
T8
T9
T10
T11
T12

Thoracic
spinal
nerves

L1
L2
L3
L4
L5

Lumbar
spinal
nerves

S1
S2
S3
S4
S5

Sacral
spinal
nerves

Posterior view

Figure CS6-4   Spinal nerves.

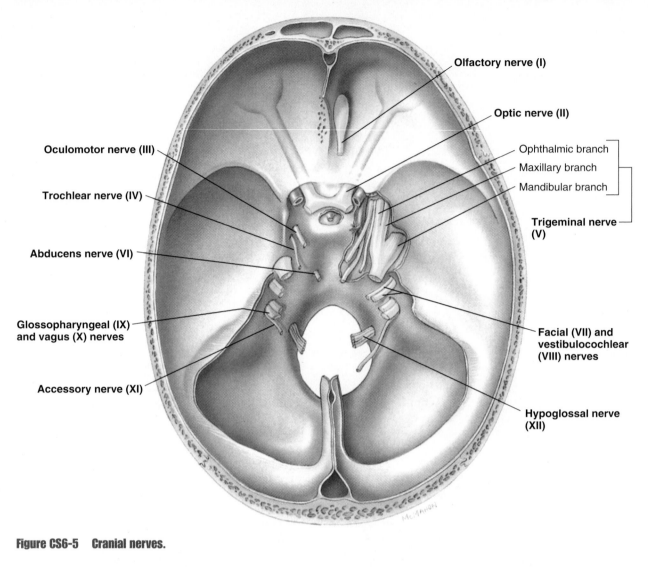

Olfactory nerve (I)

Optic nerve (II)

Oculomotor nerve (III)

Trochlear nerve (IV)

Ophthalmic branch
Maxillary branch
Mandibular branch

Trigeminal nerve (V)

Abducens nerve (VI)

Glossopharyngeal (IX) and vagus (X) nerves

Facial (VII) and vestibulocochlear (VIII) nerves

Accessory nerve (XI)

Hypoglossal nerve (XII)

Figure CS6-5   Cranial nerves.

Case 7: The Digestive System

Patient Name
Janice McClure

Address
10620 SW 72nd Court
Miami, FL 33156-5902

Situation
This elderly female had been suffering from acute abdominal pain for a few weeks before she finally presented to the Hillcrest emergency room for treatment. The emergency room physician examined her, ordered x-ray studies, admitted her, and referred her to a surgeon for evaluation. The consulting surgeon reviewed the x-ray findings, examined the patient, and discussed the options with the patient and her family. They agreed on surgery as soon as possible, which was carried out that day. An x-ray was done during the surgical procedure, and the tissues removed at surgery were submitted to pathology for gross and microscopic description and diagnosis. After an uneventful postoperative course, the patient was discharged to followup with the surgeon in two days.

Review Figure CS7-1, The Digestive System; and Figure CS7-2, Liver, Gallbladder, and Pancreas on page 96.

Student Name _____

Patient: Janice McClure

Sequence of Reports	Date Completed	Grade
History and Physical Examination	_____	_____
Request for Consultation	_____	_____
Operative Report	_____	_____
Radiology Report	_____	_____
Pathology Report	_____	_____
Discharge Summary	_____	_____

NOTE: Study the glossary for Case 7. Enter the date each report is completed in the space provided. When you have transcribed all reports, tear this sheet out, staple it to the front of the reports (in the order listed above); give completed reports to the instructor.

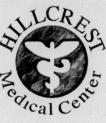

Glossary for Case 7

adenopathy (ăd″ĕ-nŏp′ah-thē)—disease (enlargement) of the glands, particularly the lymph glands

amoxicillin (ah-mŏks″ĭ-sĭl′ĭn)—generic antibiotic used against a wide variety of bacteria

ampulla (ăm-pŭl′lah)—a pouched dilatation or enlargement of a canal or duct

atypia (ā-tĭp′ē-ah)—not typical; state of being irregular

bilirubin (bĭl″ĭ-roo′bĭn)—a bile pigment circulating in plasma

calcification (kăl″sĭ-fĭ-kā′shŭn)—deposition of calcium salts in organic tissue causing the tissue to harden

cholecystitis (kō″lē-sĭs-tī′tĭs)—inflammation of the gallbladder

choledocholithiasis (kō-lĕd″ō-kō-lĭ-thī′ah-sĭs)—the condition of calculi (stones) in the common bile duct

choledocholithotomy (kō-lĕd″ō-kō-lĭ-thŏt′ō-mē)—incision of the common bile duct to remove calculi (stones)

choledochoscopy (kō-lĕd″ō-kŏs′kō-pē)—visual examination (by instrument) of the common bile duct

cholelithiasis (kō″lē-lĭ-thī′ah-sĭs)—condition (or formation) of gallstones

clips—surgical equipment; metallic devices for holding closed the edges of a wound

common bile duct—one of the ducts conveying bile from the liver to the small intestine

cranial nerves II through XII—referred to by Roman numerals, the 12 pairs of nerves connected with the brain; cranial nerve I (olfactory) is not always included in the routine physical examination

cystic artery (sĭs′tĭk ăr′tĕr-ē)—the artery that originates in the right branch of the hepatic (liver) artery and goes to the gallbladder

dentition (dĕn-tĭsh′ŭn)—the natural teeth in the dental arch

diplopia (dĭ plō′pē-ah)—double vision (seeing two images of a single object)

duodenum (dū″ō-dē′nŭm) (dū-ŏd′ĕ-nŭm)—the first portion of the small intestine

emesis (ĕm′ĕ-sĭs)—vomiting or the product derived from vomiting

eosinophils (ē″ō-sĭn′ō-fils)—cells readily stained by eosin (a red dye); part of what is reported on the differential cell count (often dictated as "eos")

ERCP—endoscopic retrograde cholangiopancreatography (an internal examination done in radiology)

expulsion—the act of expelling, driving, or forcing out

exquisite—extremely intense, sharp, as in exquisite pain or tenderness

fibrous tissue—tissue composed of or containing fibers (elongated, threadlike structures)

filling defect—any localized defect in the contour of the stomach, duodenum, or intestine as seen on the x-ray after a barium swallow or barium enema; this filling defect would be due to either a lesion or an object in the contour

flatus (flā′tŭs)—the gas or air normally in the gastrointestinal tract

follicular (fō-lĭk′ū-lăr)—pertaining to a follicle (pouchlike depression, small sac, or cavity)

frequency—the number of occurrences of a particular event, specifically urinating at short intervals due to a reduced urinary bladder capacity

gallstones—concretions (calculi) formed in the gallbladder or bile duct

GGT—abbreviation for gamma-glutamyl transpeptidase (laboratory test done on blood to check liver function)

GPT—abbreviation for glutamic-pyruvic transaminase (laboratory test done on blood to check liver function)

grossly—referring to being visible to the naked eye (grossly visible)

guarding—a spasm of muscles to minimize motion or agitation of an injured or diseased site

hernia (hĕr′nē-ah)—protrusion of all or part of an organ through the tissue normally encasing it

hesitancy—an involuntary delay (or inability) in starting the urinary stream

HIV protocol—an explicit, detailed plan regarding protection of both health care workers and patients from the human immunodeficiency virus in the workplace

indices—guides, standards, or symbols (sing., index)

interrupted 1-0 Novafil (nō′vah-fĭl)—suture material used in the fashion whereby each stitch is made with a separate piece of material; the "one-0" indicates the thickness of the thread

intraoperative cholangiogram (ĭn″trah-ŏp′ĕr-ah″tĭv kō-lăn′jē-ō-grăm″)—an x-ray of the gallbladder and bile ducts done while the patient is actually undergoing surgery

Jackson-Pratt drain—a specific tool used in surgery to draw fluid out as it forms in a cavity (sometimes dictated as J-P drain), trade name

Kocher clamp (kōk′ĕr)—a heavy, straight surgical instrument with interlocking teeth on the tip, trade name

laparoscopic cholecystectomy (lăp″ah-rō-skŏp′ĭk kō″lē-sĭs-tĕk′tō-mē)—surgical removal of the gallbladder using an instrument (laparoscope) that, when inserted, allows examination, inspection, or removal; only very small abdominal incisions are required ("lap chole" may be dictated)

lymphs (lĭmfs)—acceptable medical jargon; shortened version of lymphocytes, which are white blood cells found in blood or lymph; a part of the differential white blood cell count

mammogram (măm′ō-grăm)—the record produced by mammography (x-ray of breast)

microbiology—the science that deals with the study of microorganisms, such as algae, bacteria, fungi, protozoa, and viruses

migraine (mī′grān)—severe vascular headache

monos—acceptable medical jargon; shortened version of monocytes, which are white blood cells; a part of the differential white blood cell count

multiparous (mŭl-tĭp′ah-rŭs)—having had two or more pregnancies that resulted in birth, live or not

n.p.o. [L.]—*n*il *p*er *o*s (nothing by mouth)

needle-stick protocol—an explicit, detailed plan regarding the prevention of contaminated needle sticks to health care workers on the job

normocytic (nŏr″mō-sĭt′ĭk)—relating to or having the characteristics of a red blood cell that is normal in size, shape, and color

open cholecystectomy (kō″lē-sĭs-tĕk′tō-mē)—a surgical procedure, including an abdominal incision, for the removal of the gallbladder; it refers to surgically opening the abdomen rather than using the laparoscopic procedure

palpitations (păl″pĭ-tā′shŭnz)—sensation of an abnormally rapid heartbeat (primarily used in the plural, even if dictated in the singular)

pancreatitis (păn″krē-ah-tī′tĭs)—inflammation of the pancreas

peripheral edema (pĕ-rĭf′ĕr-al ĕ-dē′mah)—abnormally large amounts of fluid within the hands or feet; swollen hands or feet due to this fluid

peritoneal signs (pĕr″ĭ-tō-nē′ăl)—indications of disease or abnormality in the peritoneum as discovered by touching and listening over the abdominal cavity

protocol—an explicit, detailed plan of action

Provera (prō-vĕr′ah)—trade name for a drug used to treat some carcinomas as well as abnormal uterine bleeding

remote appendectomy—refers to removal of the vermiform appendix years ago, perhaps in childhood

retrograde—to go backward; moving against the usual direction of flow

Rokitansky-Aschoff sinuses (rō″kĭ-tăn′skē ăsh′ŏf)—small outpouchings of the mucosa of the gallbladder extending through the muscular layer

running sutures—in regard to surgical sutures, the opposite of interrupted sutures; continuous sutures with the stitching fastened at each end of the knot

scapular (skăp′ū-lăr)—referring to the shoulder blade or the shoulder blade area

segs—acceptable medical jargon; shortened version of *seg*mented neutrophil*s*, which are white blood cells; a part of the differential white blood cell count

sepsis (sĕp′sĭs)—toxic organisms present in the blood or other tissues

SMA—abbreviation for *s*equential *m*ultiple *a*nalyzer; a machine for automated chemical analysis of blood or serum; sometimes dictated as SMA-6 or SMA-12, etc., depending on the number of tests being done on one sample at one time

SOB—medical jargon; abbreviation for *s*hortness *o*f *b*reath

sonogram (sō′nō-grăm)—a record attained by ultrasonic scanning

stone basket—surgical instrument shaped like a basket and used to retrieve stones from the common bile duct

suspension—a state of temporary termination of liveliness, pain, or any other essential process; urinary bladder suspension refers to a procedure whereby a prolonged or fallen bladder is surgically tacked back into place

transfixed—pierced through and through with a sharp instrument

urgency—a sudden, forceful need to urinate

waxed and waned—this phrase refers to the increase of and the subsequent diminishing of an object or symptoms; like the moon waxes and wanes every month, so may symptoms wax and wane or come and go

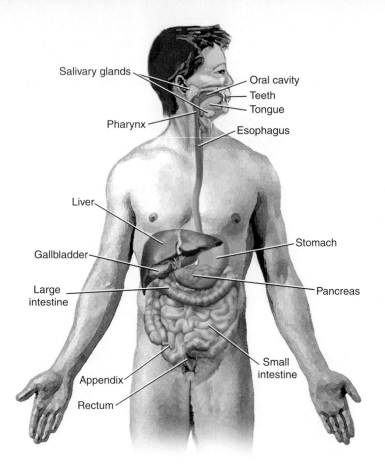

Figure CS7-1   The digestive system.

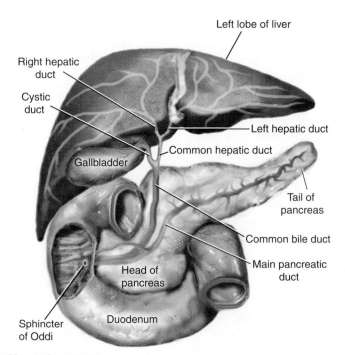

Figure CS7-2   The liver, gallbladder, and pancreas.

Case 8: The Endocrine System

ASIS AN
BA BARIU
BPD BIPA
CAT COM
CGY CEN

Patient Name
Gerald Edwards

Address
309 North Fifth Street
Miami FL 33133-4038

Situation
Gerald Edwards, a known diabetic patient, had an ulcerated area on one foot. His podiatrist referred the patient to the emergency room at Hillcrest Medical Center. The doctor in the emergency room admitted the patient and requested both the podiatrist and an ophthalmologist to consult. This was done, and the podiatrist performed necessary surgery, submitting the tissue to a pathologist for evaluation and diagnosis. The admitting doctor also ordered an MRI to be done by a radiologist who specializes in nuclear medicine. After all consultations, evaluations, and treatment were completed, the patient was discharged in improved condition. Both the podiatrist and the ophthalmologist will follow him.

Review Figure CS8-1, Bones of the Foot; and Figure CS8-2, The Endocrine System on page 99–100.

Student Name _____

Patient: Gerald Edwards

Sequence of Reports	Date Completed	Grade
History and Physical Examination	_____	_____
Request for Consultation 1	_____	_____
Request for Consultation 2	_____	_____
Radiology Report	_____	_____
Operative Report	_____	_____
Pathology Report	_____	_____
Discharge Summary	_____	_____

NOTE: Study the glossary for Case 8. Enter the date each report is completed in the space provided. When you have transcribed all reports, tear this sheet out, staple it to the front of the reports (in the order listed above); give completed reports to the instructor.

HILLCREST
Medical Center

Glossary for Case 8

acute (ah-kūt′)—a disease or condition that has a short but relatively severe course

aerobic (ā-ĕr-ō′bĭk)—having molecular oxygen present

anaerobic (ăn″ā-ĕr-ō′bĭk)—lacking molecular oxygen

Augmentin (awg-mĕn′tĭn)—antibiotic (trade name)

bacteriostatic saline (băk-tē″rē-ō-stăt′ĭk sā′lēn)—salt and water solution designed to inhibit the growth or multiplication of bacteria

beta streptococci (bā′tah strĕp″tō-kŏk′sī)—often dictated "beta strep," this refers to organisms of the genus *Streptococcus* capable of hemolyzing (dissolving) the red blood cell membrane; identified on microbacterial culture media by the clear zone produced around the bacterial colony

calor (kā′lŏr)—heat

cellulitis (sĕl″ū-lī′tĭs)—inflammation of connective tissue

Charcot disease (shăr-kō′)—neuropathic arthropathy (a joint disease)

Cipro (sĭ-prō)—antibiotic (trade name)

cuneiform (kū-nē′ĭ-fŏrm)—shaped like a wedge; a bone in the ankle

débridement [Fr.] (dā-brēd′maw) (dĭ-brēd′mĕnt)—removal of foreign material, dead or contaminated tissue from and/or adjacent to a wound or infected lesion

defervesced (dĕf″ĕr-vĕsd′)—a reduction of fever

digit (dĭj′ĭt)—a finger or toe

dorsal (dŏr′săl)—pertaining to the back

dorsalis [L.] (dŏr-sā′lĭs)—a term denoting a position closer to the back surface

dorsolateral (dŏr″sō-lăt′ĕr-ăl)—pertaining to the back and the side

dot and blot hemorrhages—a pathologic condition; tiny, round hemorrhages in the retina usually associated with diabetes mellitus

DPM—*D*octor of *P*odiatric *M*edicine

edentulous (ē-dĕn′tū-lŭs)—without teeth

encephalitis (ĕn″sĕf-ah-lī′tĭs)—inflammation of the brain

erythematous (ĕr″ĭ-thĕm′ah-tŭs)—characterized by erythema (redness of the skin)

eschar (ĕs′kăr)—a slough (necrotic tissue) formed as a result of a burn, a corrosive application, or by gangrene

gallium (găl′ē-ŭm)—a metal that has an unusually low melting point; it is a liquid at room temperature; symbol Ga

glycosylated (glī-kŏs′ĭ-lāt′ĕd)—having formed a linkage with a glycosyl (carbohydrate) group

hyperkeratotic (hī″pĕr-kĕr″ah-tŏt′ĭk)—excessive development or retention of keratin (protein of skin, hair, and nails)

I&D—*i*ncision and *d*rainage

macula (măk′ū-lah)—a stain, spot, blemish, or thickening

medial (mē′dē-ăl)—pertaining to the middle or toward the midline of the body

metatarsal (mĕt″ah-tăr′săl)—pertaining to the metatarsus (the part of the foot between the tarsus and the toes, particularly referring to the foot bones between the ankle and the toes)

mmHg—millimeters of mercury

MRI—*m*agnetic *r*esonance *i*maging (a radiologic procedure)

neovascularization (nē″ō-văs″kū-lăr-ī-zā′shŭn)—new blood vessel formation in either abnormal tissue or in abnormal position

neuropathy (nū-rŏp′ah-thē)—disease of the peripheral nervous system

NKA (NKDA)—*n*o *k*nown *a*llergies (*n*o *k*nown *d*rug allergies)

Nu Gauze (nū′gawz)—products used in surgery and for wound care (trade name)

osseous (ŏs′ē-ŭs)—composed of or pertaining to the nature or quality of bone; bony

osteomyelitis (ŏs″tē-ō-mī″ĕ-lī′tĭs)—inflammation of bone caused by a pyogenic organism

plantar (plăn′tăr)—pertaining to the sole of the foot

retinopathy (rĕt″ĭ-nŏp′ah-thē)—disease of the retina

sanguinopurulent (săng″gwĭ-nō-pū′rū-lĕnt)—containing both blood and pus

T&A—*t*onsils and *a*denoids, or *t*onsillectomy and *a*denoidectomy

tabes dorsalis [L.] (tā′bēz dŏr-sā′lĭs)—a degeneration of the dorsal column of the spinal cord and of the sensory nerve trunks

tarsal (tahr′săl)—pertaining to the instep; any of the seven bones of the tarsus (ankle)

tendinous (tĕn′dĭ-nŭs)—pertaining to a tendon

tie-over dressing—a dressing placed over a skin graft and tied on by sutures that have been left long enough for that purpose

Trental (trĕn′tăl)—a drug used to treat peripheral vascular disease (trade name)

tympanic (tĭm-păn′ĭk)—pertaining to the tympanic membrane (eardrum) that separates the middle from the external ear; sometimes dictated TM

Unasyn (ū′nă-sĭn)—antibiotic (trade name)

venous (vē′nŭs)—pertaining to a vein or veins

vitreous (vĭt′rē-ŭs)—glasslike, pertains to the jellylike mass that fills the cavity of the eye

Webril padding (wĕb′rĭl)—material used during surgery to protect the skin of the extremity under a tourniquet (trade name)

Xeroflo (zē′rō-flō)—gauze dressing (trade name)

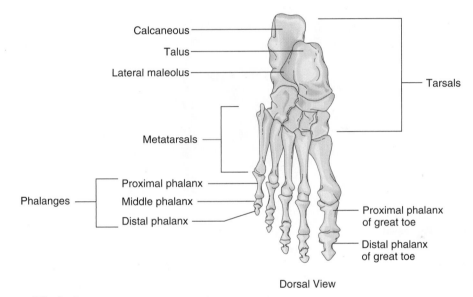

Dorsal View

Figure CS8-1   Bones of the foot.

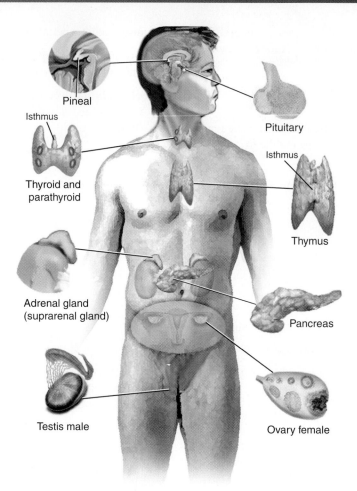

ASIS ANT
BA BARIU
BPD BIPA
CAT COM
CGY CEN

Patient Name
Mark Thomas

Address
9038 SW 45th Terrace
South Miami, FL 33165-5912

Situation
This young man had been suffering from shortness of breath; with his history of lymphoma he finally went to see a physician, a surgeon, who admitted him to Hillcrest. In the subsequent workup, the patient's oncologist was notified of the readmission, and radiology was involved in a special study. After the planned surgical procedure the tissue removed was submitted to pathology for evaluation and diagnosis. On discharge the patient's shortness of breath was improved, and he was scheduled to go back on chemotherapy. He is to have a GI workup as an outpatient.

Review Figure CS9-1, The Lymphatic System, and Figure CS9-2, Structure of the Lymph Node, on pages 104–105.

Student Name _____

Patient: Mark Thomas

Sequence of Reports	Date Completed	Grade
History and Physical Examination	_____	_____
Operative Report	_____	_____
Pathology Report	_____	_____
Radiology Report	_____	_____
Discharge Summary	_____	_____

NOTE: Study the glossary for Case 9. Enter the date each report is completed in the space provided. When you have transcribed all reports, tear this sheet out, staple it to the front of the reports (in the order listed above); give completed reports to the instructor.

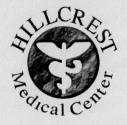

Glossary for Case 9

abdominal (ăb-dŏm′ĭ-năl)—pertaining to the abdomen

Adriamycin (ā″drē-ah-mī′sĭn)—antibiotic used only in chemotherapy (trade name)

amiodarone (ah-mē-ō′-dah-rŏn″)—antiarrhythmic drug (generic)

anergy panel (ăn′ĕr-jē)—a group of substances to which a patient's allergic susceptibility is tested

apex (a′pĕks)—a general term used to designate the top of a body, organ, or part

arrhythmia (ah-rĭth′mē-ah)—any variation from the normal rhythm of the heartbeat

arteriole (ăr-tē′rē-ōl)—a minute arterial branch

atraumatic (ā″traw-măt′ĭk)—not inflicting or causing damage or injury; not damaged or injured; without trauma

atropine (ăt′rō-pēn)—generic drug used preoperatively as a muscle relaxer and to inhibit salivation and secretions; it has other uses, too

axilla (ăk-sĭl′ah)—armpit (pl. axillae)

bibasilar rales (bī′bās′ĭ-lăr rahls)—crackling sounds heard in the bases of both lungs

bronchomalacia (brŏng″kō-mah-lā′shē-ah)—degeneration of elastic and connective tissue of bronchi and trachea

bronchoscope (brŏng′kō-skōp)—instrument with which to examine the bronchi

bronchospasm (brŏng′kō-spăzm)—spasmodic contraction of the smooth muscle of the bronchi

cardiac (kăr′dē-ăk)—pertaining to the heart

carina (kah-rī′nah)—a ridgelike structure

costophrenic (kŏs″tō-frĕn′ĭk)—pertaining to the ribs and diaphragm

cytology (sī-tŏl′ō-jē)—the study of cells

diabetes mellitus (dī″ah-bē′tēz mĕ-lī′tŭs) (dī″ah-bē′tēz mĕl′lĭ-tŭs)—a metabolic disease due to an abnormality of insulin; diabetes is associated with multiple complications of various organs and systems

DLCO—*d*iffusing capacity of the *l*ung for carbon monoxide (*CO*)

dorsalis pedis [L.] (dor-sā′lĭs pē′dĭs)—a term denoting a position closer to the back surface of the foot

Ecotrin (ĕk′ō-trĭn)—nonsteroidal anti-inflammatory drug (trade name)

epigastric (ĕp″ĭ-găs′trĭk)—pertaining to the epigastrium

epigastrium (ĕp″ĭ-găs′trē-ŭm)—the upper middle region of the abdomen

esophageal reflux (ĕ-sŏf″ah-jē′ăl rē′flŭks)—a backward flow or regurgitation of stomach contents

FEV₁ or FEV1—*f*orced *e*xpiratory *v*olume in one second (part of the pulmonary function tests)

FVC—*f*orced *v*ital *c*apacity (part of the pulmonary function tests)

gait (gāt)—the manner or style of walking

gastritis (găs-trī′tĭs)—inflammation of the stomach

heaves (hēvz)—a respiratory disturbance characterized by partially forced expiration

holosystolic murmur (hō″lō-sĭs-tŏl′ĭk mŭr′mŭr)—heart sound heard over the entire systole, or the period of contraction; also called pansystolic murmur

HTN—*h*yper*ten*sion

hypokinesis (hī″pō-kī-nē′sĭs)—abnormally decreased mobility

IM—*i*ntra*m*uscularly; within the muscle(s)

infrahilar (ĭn″frah-hī′lăr)—below the hilum (a depression or pit)

jugular venous (jŭg″ū-lăr vē′nŭs)—referring to the jugular vein in the neck

Lasix (lā′sĭks)—trade name for a drug used to manage edema and/or hypertension

lavage (lah-vahzh′)—irrigation of an organ

LVEF—*l*eft *v*entricular *e*jection *f*raction (a cardiac term)

macrophage (măk′rō-fāj)—large cells with a round or indented nucleus

morphine (mŏr′fēn)—generic drug used as a narcotic; pain medication

MUGA—*mu*ltiple *g*ated *a*cquisition (scan), a radiologic procedure

naris (năr′ĭs)—one of the openings of the nasal cavity; a nostril (pl. nares)

nebulizer (nĕb′ū-līz″ĕr)—an atomizer; a device for throwing a spray

necrosis (nĕ-krō′sĭs)—cell death

non-Hodgkin lymphoma (lĭm-fō′mah)—a group of malignant lymphomas; a neoplasm arising from the lymphatics; the most common manifestation is the painless enlargement of one or more lymph nodes

oximetry (ŏk-sĭm′ĕ-trē)—an instrument (oximeter) used to determine the oxygen saturation of arterial blood

Pepcid (pĕp′sĭd)—blocker drug to heal ulcers (trade name)

PFT, PFTs—*p*ulmonary *f*unction *t*est or *t*ests

pneumothorax (nū″mō-thō′răks)—an accumulation of air or gas in the pleural space, which is the serous membrane that surrounds the lungs and lines the thoracic cavity

PPD—*p*urified *p*rotein *d*erivative (of tuberculin); skin test for tuberculosis

Propacet (prō′pă-sĕt)—a pain medication (trade name)

RDW—*r*ed (cell) *d*istribution *w*idth (a laboratory term)

S/P—*s*tatus *p*ost; used to indicate the patient's condition after a procedure, e.g., status post appendectomy, status post chemotherapy, status post MVA

sternal (stĕr′năl)—pertaining to the sternum

Tenormin (tĕn′ŏr-mĭn)—drug used to treat angina and hypertension; also used for migraine headaches (trade name)

thrill (thrĭl)—a vibration sensation felt by the examiner on palpation of (feeling) the body; often a cardiac term

transbronchial (trăns-brŏng′kē-ăl)—referring to across the bronchus

Vasotec (vā′zō-tĕk)—inhibitor drug used for hypertension (trade name)

Ventolin (vĕn′tō-lĭn)—a drug used in asthma and other respiratory diseases to reverse airway obstruction (trade name)

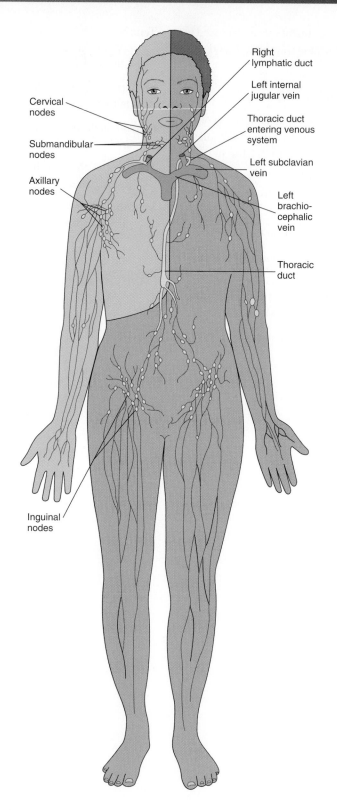

Figure CS9-1   The lymphatic system.

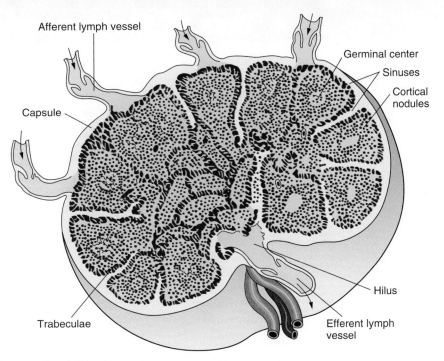

Figure CS9-2 Structure of the lymph node.

ANYL
RIUM
BIPAR
COMP
ENTI

Case 10: The Respiratory System

Patient Name
Scott Chandler

Address
14302 Briarbend
Kay Biscayne, FL 33149-6747

Situation

This elderly patient found himself in respiratory distress and was brought by ambulance to Hillcrest emergency room early one morning. The emergency room physicians together with a pulmonary/thoracic surgeon performed emergency surgery. The radiology department did serial chest x-rays to determine whether the patient's lung remained expanded. Due to a worsening in the patient's respiratory status, the surgeon performed a second procedure; radiology continued to keep a close check on his chest and lungs. After continued complications and significant deterioration in the patient's condition, the pulmonary/thoracic surgeon was requested to assess the patient. He recommended transfer to Forrest General Medical Center for more complicated surgery. The patient was transferred to Forrest General for further evaluation and care.

Review Figure CS10-1, The Respiratory System, and Figure CS10-2, Structure of the Lungs, on pages 108–109.

Student Name _____

Patient: Scott Chandler

Sequence of Reports	Date Completed	Grade
History and Physical Examination	_____	_____
Operative Report 1	_____	_____
Radiology Report 1	_____	_____
Radiology Report 2	_____	_____
Operative Report 2	_____	_____
Radiology Report 3	_____	_____
Request for Consultation	_____	_____
Discharge Summary	_____	_____

NOTE: Study the glossary for Case 10. Enter the date each report is completed in the space provided. When you have transcribed all reports, tear this sheet out, staple it to the front of the reports (in the order listed above); give completed reports to the instructor.

HILLCREST
Medical Center

Glossary for Case 10

ablation (ăb-lā′shŭn)—to separate, detach, or remove an organ or tissue, especially by surgical means

anesthetize (ah-nĕs′thĕ-tīz)—to put under the influence of anesthetics—drugs or agents used to abolish the sensation of pain

aorta (ā-ŏr′tah)—the main trunk of the arterial system, conveying blood from the heart

benzoin (bĕn′zoin)—a topical antiseptic, generic

bronchodilator (brŏng″kō-dī-lā′tŏr)—stretching or expanding the air passages of the lungs or a medicinal agent that produces such results

bronchopleural (brŏng″kō-ploor′ăl)—pertaining to a bronchus and the pleura

cannula (kăn′ū-lah)—a tube for insertion into a duct or cavity

catheter (kăth′ĕ-tĕr)—a tubular, flexible instrument (metal or rubber) for either withdrawing fluids or introducing fluids into a body cavity or vessel

ciprofloxacin (sĭp″rō-flŏx-ă-cĭn)—generic name for a broad-spectrum antibiotic

COPD—*c*hronic *o*bstructive *p*ulmonary *d*isease

decubitus (dē-kū′bĭ-tŭs)—the position assumed in lying down (decubitus position, decubitus ulcers)

emergent (ē-mĕr′jĕnt)—pertaining to an emergency

emphysema (ĕm″fĭ-sē′mah)—a pathologic accumulation of air in tissues or organs, which causes abnormal swelling of body tissues

fistula (fĭs′tū-lah)—an abnormal passageway (often created by a surgical procedure) usually between two internal organs or leading from an internal organ to the surface of the body, e.g., colostomy

hemithorax (hēm″ē-thō′răks)—one side of the chest

hemostat (hē′mō-stăt)—a small surgical clamp for constricting a blood vessel

HJR—*h*epato*j*ugular *r*eflux (a GI term)

hypertension (hī″pĕr-tĕn′shŭn)—persistently high arterial blood pressure

ichthyosis (ĭk″thē-ō′sĭs)—dryness and fishlike scaling of the skin

loculate (lŏk′ū-lāt)—divided into loculi (cavities)

loculus (lŏk′ū-lŭs)—a small space or cavity (pl. loculi)

marked—noticeable; to an extreme

PCO₂—*p*artial pressure (or tension) of carbon dioxide or CO_2 (done on blood gas studies)

percutaneous (pĕr″kū-tā′nē-ŭs)—performed through the skin

pH—hydrogen ion concentration in urine, blood, and other body fluids (neutral = 7.00; more than 7.00 is alkaline; less than 7.00 is acidic). NOTE: Always pH, even at beginning of sentence.

Pleur-Evac system (suction or tube) (ploor′ē-văk)—thoracic drainage system (equipment), trade name

pleurodesis (ploo-rō-dē′sĭs)—the production of adhesions between the parietal and the visceral pleura

PO₂—*p*artial pressure (tension) of oxygen or O_2 (a blood gas term)

portable chest—medical jargon pertaining to the equipment used and the process of obtaining a chest x-ray outside of the radiology department

Proventil (prō-vĕn′tĭl)—bronchodilator (trade name)

Pseudomonas aeruginosa (soo″dō-mō′năs ĕ″rū-gĭn-ō′sah)—the type of bacterial species of the genus, and the only one pathogenic for humans, made up of microorganisms that produce the blue-green pigment that gives the color to "blue pus" observed in certain suppurative infections

radiograph (rā′dē-o-grăf″)—film produced by radiography, commonly called an x-ray

resolution—the subsidence or disappearance of a pathologic condition

Rocephin (rō-sĕf′ĭn)—antibiotic (trade name)

sclerotherapy (sklĕ″rō-thĕr′ah-pē)—treatment involving the injection of a sclerosing or hardening solution into vessels or tissues

stat (stăt)—abbreviation for [L.] statim (immediately); largely misused, it is meant to convey a life or death emergency

Streptococcus (strĕp″tō-kŏk′ŭs)—bacteria growing in chains found in human mouth and intestine; sometimes they can cause disease

subtherapeutic (sŭb″thĕr′ah-pū′tĭk)—a less than therapeutic level, usually referring to the blood level of a particular drug or medication

tachycardia (tăk″ē-kăr′dē-ah)—fast heart rate

Theo-Dur (thē′ō-dŭr)—theophylline, a bronchodilator used in patients with asthma or COPD (trade name)

theophylline (thē-ŏf′ĭ-lĭn)—a smooth muscle relaxant, used chiefly for its bronchodilator effect

thoracic (thō-răs′ĭk)—pertaining to the chest

thoracostomy (thō″rah-kŏs′tō-mē)—surgical creation of an opening in the thorax (chest wall) for the purpose of drainage

thoracotomy (thō″rah-kŏt′ō-mē)—surgical incision into the thorax

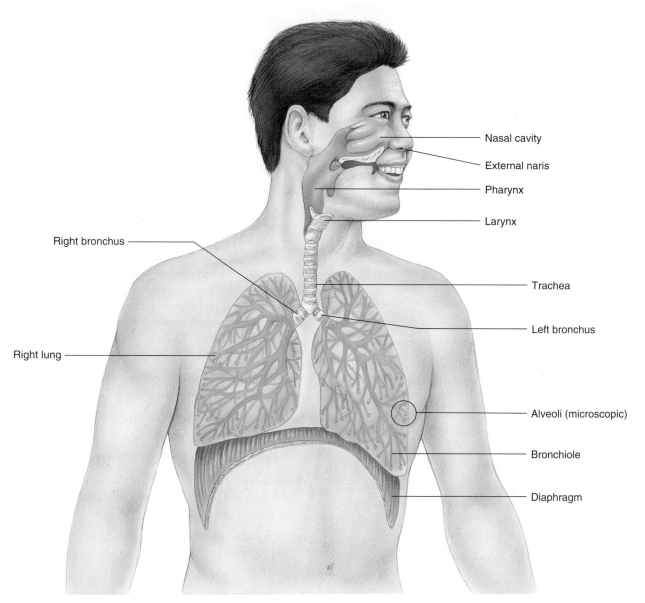

Figure CS10-1   The respiratory system.

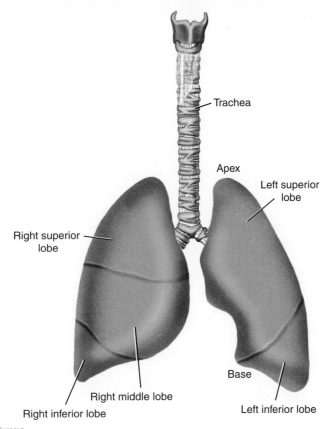

Trachea

Apex

Left superior
lobe

Right superior
lobe

Right middle lobe

Base

Right inferior lobe

Left inferior lobe

Figure CS10-2 Structure of the lungs.

Section 5
Quali-Care Clinic

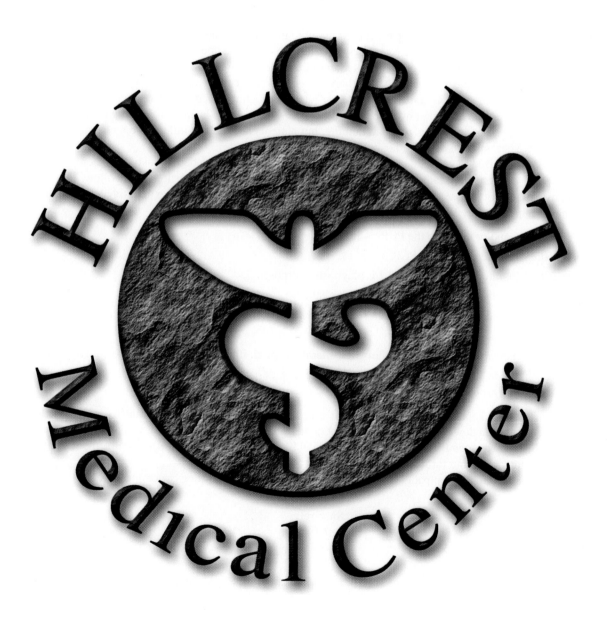

You will be transcribing outpatient medical reports for Quali-Care Clinic, a medical facility housed in a freestanding office building adjacent to Hillcrest Medical Center and containing the offices of physicians and health care providers from 12 different medical specialties. Those in the specialties of Family Practice and Internal Medicine act as primary care physicians (PCPs) who see their patients on a regular basis, paying close attention to their overall well-being and referring them to specialists or to Hillcrest Medical Center for further evaluation and treatment as necessary. (NOTE: PCPs for female patients include Gynecology and Obstetrics.)

You will be transcribing 25 outpatient reports that relate to these medical specialty areas. These reports demonstrate variations in style, format, and content common to the dictating habits of the originators of medical records—habits usually learned while in medical school. Model Report Form 9 (page 35) shows a model HPIP report (history, physical, impression, plan) and Model Report Form 10 (page 36) shows a model SOAP report (subjective, objective, assessment, plan). These two formats or variations thereof are the mainstay of the physicians' outpatient medical record (chart) on each patient. The SOAP format is less formal and generally used in doctors' chart notes. Each physician personalizes a format using a preferred style. Correspondence is introduced in these reports, which is one way PCPs and consultants communicate with each other. See Model Report Form 11 on page 37 for an example.

Included in a medical record would be patient demographic information, the next of kin, what to do in case of emergency, laboratory and x-ray results, and vital signs written in at each visit. The doctor may dictate chart notes after each patient visit and telephone call *or* these notes may be handwritten. Elderly or very ill patients or families may be counseled regarding a living will, a directive to physicians, or otherwise asked to indicate their wishes should a terminal situation exist. This may be referred to as "DNR" status or a "no code" status, which means do not resuscitate (DNR) should cardiac or respiratory failure occur, and do not allow hospital or emergency personnel to institute lifesaving measures (like a "Code Blue"). There are many variations in this type of planning, but patients and their families have the right and the responsibility to state their wishes and to have them honored.

When a patient is referred to a specialist, special examinations or procedures, both invasive and noninvasive, may occur. If all attempts to cure a patient fail using outpatient measures, then inpatient measures must follow. This involves admission to a hospital, either Hillcrest, the adjacent 400-bed-transplant facility, burn center, and rehabilitation unit.

In summary, outpatient care is done on the following levels.

1. Telephone calls and/or letters to the PCP
2. Scheduled appointments with the PCP
3. Requests for laboratory tests and x-rays for diagnostic purposes
4. Referral to a specialist (or consultant) for further evaluation and treatment
5. Treatment in the specialist's (or consultant's) office with more advanced, noninvasive procedures
6. Invasive procedures that include surgery
7. Transfer to Hillcrest Medical Center or Forrest General Hospital, if necessary, for further evaluation and treatment
8. Aftercare to include physical therapy, occupational therapy, nursing home care—either skilled (short term) or custodial (long term)—with appropriate followup by the original PCP

Extensive records are kept at each level of patient care, and this involves dictation and transcription. Remember, *legally,* what was not written down or transcribed was not done. MTs create records that are vital to patient care and are legal documents subject to subpoena. They also create a medical history that is the basis for reimbursement from third-party payers (insurance companies) and for research purposes.

We hope that transcribing the outpatient reports proves to be a valuable learning experience.

Sincerely,

Allison Poole

Allison Poole, CMT, RHIA
Director, Information Management Department

Quali-Care Clinic Outpatient Report Log

Student Name _____

Enter the date of completion below for each Quali-Care Clinic outpatient report or letter. When completed, give this sheet or a copy of it to your instructor along with your work. (The log may be adapted as needed.)

Report Number/Patient Name/Report Type	Date Completed	Grade
QC 1, Nancy Lee Beltran/GYN Operative Report		
QC 2, Nancy Lee Beltran/Pathology Report		
QC 3, Nancy Lee Beltran/Cytology Report		
QC 4, Betty Crane/Oncology Consult		
QC 5, Jimmy McGann/Infectious Disease SOAP Note		
QC 6, Doug Peters/Pulmonology Procedure Note		
QC 7, Jana Stevens/Oncology Consult		
QC 8, Jana Stevens/Correspondence		
QC 9, Jorge Romero/Infectious Disease Consult		
QC 10, Carlos Ledesma/Pediatrics—Emergency Center Report		
QC 11, Harold Rivers/Internal Medical History and Physical		
QC 12, Barbara Ann Richards/Psychiatry Consult		
QC 13, Maggie Ricks/Radiology—Echocardiogram Report		
QC 14, Leon Markowitz/Radiology—Colonoscopy Procedure Note		
QC 15, Maggie Ricks/Radiology—CT Scan of Abdomen		
QC 16, Otto Werner Valtin/Infectious Disease HPIP Note		
QC 17, Doris Dean/Radiology—Mammogram and CT Scan of Abdomen		
QC 18, Sterling Peak/Oncology Consult		
QC 19, Sterling Peak/Correspondence		
QC 20, John J. Crawford/Pulmonology—Sleep Study		
QC 21, Leslie Arispe/Psychiatry Consult		
QC 22, Emily Pickens/ Radiology—MRI		
QC 23, B. Christine Anello/Pediatrics—Emergency Center Report		
QC 24, Sabar Samaan/Hematology Consult		
QC 25, Sabar Samaan/Correspondence		

Outpatient Reports

This section contains a brief explanation of each patient's reason for receiving outpatient medical care at Quali-Care Clinic. A glossary of medical terms found in each report is included.

REPORT 1: GYNECOLOGY OPERATIVE REPORT

Nancy Lee Beltran was admitted to One-Day Surgery at Quali-Care Clinic for laparoscopic removal of her fallopian tubes and ovaries due to an ovarian mass. She also had adhesions that required lysis. The patient was discharged from One-Day Surgery after four hours in postanesthesia recovery (PAR). Office followup was scheduled. Copies of her surgical record were sent to her family doctor and to the surgeon's office. See Figure QC1-1, Structures of the Female Reproductive System, on page 116.

GLOSSARY		
Word	**Phonetic Prounciation**	**Definition**
1-0 Vicryl	(vī′krĭl)	trade name for polyglactin 910, a suture material; 1-0 refers to the width of the suture material
3-0 Vicryl		see above; this 3-0 suture material is finer than 1-0
abdominopelvic adhesive disease	(ăb-dŏm″ĭ-nō-pĕl′vĭk)	adhesions located in the abdominal and pelvic cavities
adhesiolysis	(ăd-hē″zē-ō li′sis)	separation, destruction of adhesions
ambulatory	(ăm′bū-lă-tŏr-ē)	able to walk
bipolar cauterized	(kaw′tĕr-ized)	electrocautery with a device having two probes or needles, between which current flows through tissue
catheter	(kăth′ĕ-tĕr)	a tubular, flexible instrument for withdrawing fluids or introducing fluids into a body cavity or a vessel
cul-de-sac [Fr.]	(kŭl′dĕ-sahk′)	a blind pouch
Davidson grasper		trade name for equipment used in surgery to grasp tissue, allowing it to be held in place while it is being cut prior to its removal
diagnostic laparoscopy	(lăp″ah-rŏs′kō-pē)	inserting a scope into the abdomen for diagnostic purposes
EndoCatch		a bag used in endoscopic surgery into which an organ or object is placed so that it can be removed through one of the tiny abdominal incisions (trade name)
Endoloop		trade name for a disposable suture ligature instrument
epinephrine	(ĕp″ĭ-nĕf′rin)	generic drug used as a vasoconstrictor, cardiac stimulant, and bronchodilator; adrenaline
fascia	(făsh′ē-ah)	supportive layer of thin connective tissue within the muscles and/or organs of the body
general endotracheal (anesthesia)	(ĕn″dō-trā′kē-ăl)	anesthesia in which a tube is inserted into the trachea so that the entire body can be anesthetized (put to sleep)
Hasson cannula	(hăsŏn′ kăn′ū-lah)	trade name for a tube that is inserted into a duct or cavity

	GLOSSARY	
Word	**Phonetic Prounciation**	**Definition**
hemostasis	(hē″mō-stā′sĭs)	the arrest of bleeding due to a physiological process (vasoconstriction and coagulation) or by surgical means
infundibulopelvic ligament	(ĭn″fŭn-dĭb″ū-lō-pĕl′vĭk)	the suspensory ligament of the ovary
insufflated	(ĭn″sŭ-flā′tĕd)	a powder, vapor, gas, or air that has been blown into a body cavity
laparoscopic lysis	(lăp″ah-rō-skŏp′ĭk lī′sĭs)	separation of adhesions with instruments inserted through separate small incisions while observing through a laparoscope
lithotomy position	(lĭ-thŏt′ō-mē)	position of the body while lying on the back with legs lifted and separated, appropriate for GYN surgery
Marcaine	(mahr-kān′)	trade name for local, injectable anesthetic agent
monopolar cautery	(mŏn′ō-pō″lĕr kaw′ter-ē)	burning using an instrument with a single electrical pole
morcellated	(mōr-sĕ-lāt′ĕd)	piecemeal removal of a tumor or solid tissue
No. 1 PDS		*polydioxanone sutures*, No. 1 being the size of the suture material
No. 1 Vicryl stay sutures		trade name for polyglactin 910, No. 1 being the size of the suture material; stay sutures are heavy, absorbable sutures used to reinforce wound closure
normal pelvic anatomy		the condition of no abnormalities having been found on examination of the pelvic cavity
omental abdominal wall adhesions	(ō-měn′tăl)	adhesions located in the omentum, which is a free fold of the peritoneum that connects the stomach to other adjacent visceral organs
pedicles	(pěd′ĭ-k′ls)	footlike or stemlike structures
peritoneum	(pěr′ĭ-tō-nē′ŭm)	the serous membrane lining the abdominal walls and investing the viscera
prepped and draped		medical jargon meaning that the surgical field has been shaved, scrubbed, draped with sterile drapes, and otherwise prepared for the upcoming procedure; "prepped" is short for "prepared" and is acceptable for use in medical transcription
psoas muscle	(sō′ăs)	one of two muscles of the loin that connect the spinal column and the thighbone
round ligament		round ligament (of uterus) is in the upper part of the uterus
Rx		abbreviation for prescription
salpingo-oophorectomy	(săl-pĭng″gō-ō″ŏf-ō-rĕk′tō-mē)	surgical removal of both a uterine tube and an ovary
serous fluid	(sēr′ŭs)	fluid having the nature of serum; fluid between two layers comprising a serous membrane

	GLOSSARY	
Word	**Phonetic Prounciation**	**Definition**
serous papillary cystadenoma	(păp′ĭ-lair″ē sĭs″tăd-ĕ-nō′mă)	a tumor distended by fluid
sharp and blunt dissection		dissection occurring by cutting tissue with a sharp instrument, then by separating tissue along natural lines without cutting; takes a singular verb
sponge stick		a surgical sponge used to blot tissue within a wound
suprapubic	(soo″prah-pū′bĭk)	situated superior to the pubic arch
Trendelenburg (position)	(trĕn′dĕ-lĕn-bĕrg)	patient lying supine on the operating table, with the head tilted down at 30 to 40 degrees, so that the head is lower than the feet
umbilical port	(ŭm-bĭl′ĭ-kăl)	port inserted in the umbilicus to provide an opening
umbilicus	(ŭm-bĭl′ĭ-kŭs)	the navel
unipolar cautery		burning using an instrument with a single electric pole

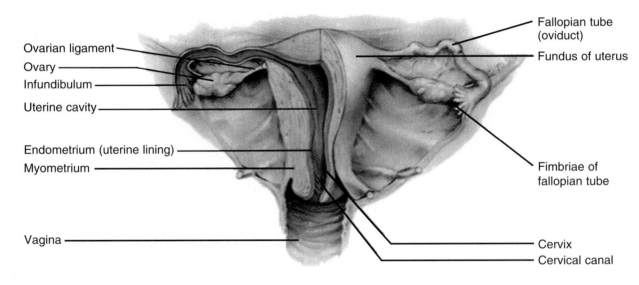

Figure QC1-1   Structures of the Female Reproductive System

REPORT 2: PATHOLOGY REPORT

Ms. Beltran's surgical specimens were sent for histologic and cytologic evaluation. Frozen section diagnosis had been made during the surgical procedure. Her final pathologic diagnosis was benign. See Figure QC2-1, Comparison of Cells, on page 118.

GLOSSARY		
Word	**Phonetic Prounciation**	**Definition**
aggregate	(ăg′rah-gĕt)	crowded or clustered together
atrophic ovarian stroma	(ă-trōf′ĭk ō-vār′ē-ăn strō′mă)	a wasting away of the ovarian supportive tissue
benign serous papillary cystadenoma	(sēr′ŭs păp′ĭ-lair″ē sĭs″tăd-ĕ-nō′mă)	a nonmalignant type of glandular tumor distended by fluid
bilateral salpingo-oophorectomy	(săl-pĭng″gō-ō″ŏf-ō-rĕk′tō-mē)	surgical removal of both uterine tubes and ovaries
ciliated cytoplasm	(sĭl′ē-āt-ĕd sī′tō-plăz″ĕm)	a fringe of hair (cilia) at the site of the cell that has most of the chemical activities
columnar epithelium	(ĕp″ĭ-thē′lē-ŭm)	cells covering the external surface of the body that are composed of tall, prismatic cells
corpora albicantia	(kŏr′pō-rah ăl′bĭ-kan″shē-ah)	white fibrous tissue that replaces the corpus luteum, a mass of yellow tissue formed in the ovary immediately after ovulation
cuboidal epithelium	(kū-boi′dăl)	cube-shaped cells lining the vessels and other small cavities within the anatomy
cystic follicles	(sĭs′tĭk fŏl′ĭ-k′ls)	saclike structures that resemble cysts
cytology	(sī tol′ō-jē)	the study of cells
cytoplasmic ciliation	(sī″tō-plăz′mĭk sĭl′ē-ā″shŭn)	a fringe of hair (cilia) at the site of the cell that has most of the chemical activities
excrescence	(ĕks-krĕs′ĕns)	an abnormal or disfiguring outgrowth
fallopian tube	(fă-lō′pē-ăn)	also known as uterine tube or oviduct; one of two tubes that carry ova from the ovaries to the uterus
fibrotic wall	(fī-brŏt′ĭk)	a wall of tissue that is repairing or replacing the essential elements of an organ
fimbria	(fĭm′brē-ah)	fingerlike extensions at the opening of a fallopian tube
fimbriated end		the end having fingerlike extensions
formalin	(for′mă-lĭn)	an aqueous solution of formaldehyde used to preserve tissue removed at surgery for pathologic evaluation
lumen	(loo′mĕn)	the cavity or channel within a vessel
malignancy		a cancerous tumor
mitotic activity	(mī-tŏt′ĭk)	a complex process of cell division
neoplasia	(nē″ō-plā′zē-ah)	a new, abnormal formation of cell tissue
nuclear atypicality		a nucleus with an abnormal formation
oophorectomy	(ōōforek′tō-mē)	excision of an ovary
ovarian stroma	(ō-vār′ē-ăn strō′mah)	the supporting tissue of an ovary

GLOSSARY		
Word	**Phonetic Prounciation**	**Definition**
papillary excrescences		nipplelike structures that are abnormal outgrowths of morbid origin
papillations	(păp′ĭ-lā″shunz)	small, nipple-shaped structures
pathology	(păth′ŏl-ō-gē)	study of disease
preliminary fixation		initially placing tissue in a fixative prior to preparation of same for pathologic examination
salpingectomy	(sal″pĭn-jĕk′tō-mē)	removal of a uterine tube
tubo-epithelial structures	(too-bō″-ĕp″ĭ-thē-lē-ăl)	structures of fallopian tube and skin
tubo-ovarian complex	(too-bō″-ō-vār′e-ăn)	the combined fallopian tube and ovary
tufts		small clusters of hairs

Figure QC2-1   Comparison of Normal Cells to Cancerous Cells (Courtesy of National Cancer Society)

REPORT 3: CYTOLOGY REPORT

The fluid sent for cytologic examination from Ms. Beltran's procedure was tested and found to be benign. Copies of her histology and cytology reports were sent to her family doctor and to her surgeon. See Figure QC 3-1, Endocervical Smear.

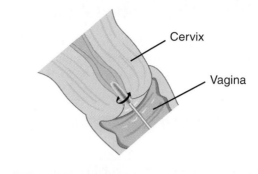

Figure QC3-1   Endocervical Smear

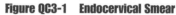

Word	Phonetic Prounciation	Definition
admixed lymphocytes	(lĭm′fō-sīts)	cells found in lymph and lymphoid tissues that are mixed together
cell block		a mass of cells, compacted and embedded in paraffin for histologic examination
Cytospin	(sī′tō-spĭn)	trade name for equipment used in histology and cytology departments to prepare (fix) specimens for microscopic examination and diagnosis
Diff-Quik	(dĭf-qwĭk)	trade name for a product used in fixing specimens, as is done in the histology and cytology sections of pathology departments
eosin	(ē′ō-sĭn)	a rose-colored stain
hematoxylin	(hē″mă-tŏk′sĭ-lĭn)	a stain used to fix histology specimens; H&E (hematoxylin and eosin) staining is standard
luteinized cells	(loo″tē-ĭn′īzed)	after ovulation, the ovarian follicles become hypertrophied and lipids accumulate in the follicles
mesothelial cells	(měz″ō-thē′lē-ăl)	the middle layer of cells that line the serous membranes of the peritoneum, pleura, and pericardium
Papanicolaou technique	(pă″pĕ-nĭ″kō-lăo″oo)	a test used to detect abnormal cells, often referred to as a Pap smear; created by George N. Papanicolaou, Greek physician, 1883–1962
proteinaceous background	(prō″tēn-ā′shŭs)	when observing a specimen fixed on a glass slide under a microscope, the background appears to be filled with protein

GLOSSARY

REPORT 4: ONCOLOGY CONSULT

Betty Crane was referred from the Hillcrest emergency room for an oncology consult after presenting with bloody nipple discharge and the actual loss of her right nipple. The patient was examined, biopsied, and further workup was planned to rule out breast cancer. A copy of the report was sent to the general surgeon who had referred her to oncology. See Figures QC4-1A and B, The Mammary Glands, on page 121.

GLOSSARY		
Word	**Phonetic Prounciation**	**Definition**
atraumatic inflicting	(ā″traw-măt′ĭk)	no damage or injury; not damaged or injured
auscultation	(aws″kŭl-tā′shŭn)	the act of listening for sounds within the body
axillae	(ăk-sĭl′ē)	armpits (sing. axilla)
bacterial colonization		when bacteria are present in such numbers as to form a colony
bowel sounds		abdominal sounds caused by peristaltic action of the intestine
CA 15-3		an antigen (breast cancer tumor marker)
calcifications		the process by which organic tissue becomes hardened by a deposit of calcium salts
CBC		abbreviation for *complete blood count* (laboratory test done on venous blood)
cerebral cancer	(sĕ-rē′brăl)	a malignancy of the cerebrum or main portion of the brain
chem-18		chemical profile (laboratory tests) resulting in 18 different values, done on either blood or serum
clot		coagulation of blood or lymph; an insoluble mass
clubbing		change (broadening) of the soft tissues around the ends of the fingers or toes; the nails are abnormally curved and shiny
congestive heart failure		condition of impaired ability of the heart to pump blood
cyanosis	(sī″ah-nō′sĭs)	a bluish discoloration
diabetes	(dī″ah-bē′tēz)	a metabolic disease due to an abnormality of insulin
edema	(ĕ-dē′mah)	abnormal accumulation of fluid in the intercellular tissue spaces of the body, resulting in swelling
emphysema	(ĕm″fĭ-sē′mah)	a pathologic accumulation of air in tissues, especially the lungs
extraocular muscles intact		unimpaired muscles that lie adjacent to but outside the eyeball
glucose		sugar
Hct		abbreviation for hematocrit (red blood cells); sometimes dictated "crit"
HEENT		*h*ead, *e*yes, *e*ars, *n*ose, *t*hroat
hepatosplenomegaly	(hĕp″ah-tō-splē′nō-mĕg′ah-lē)	enlargement of the liver and spleen
Hgb		abbreviation for hemoglobin (oxygen-carrying pigment in red blood cells)
HPI		*h*istory of *p*resent *i*llness
hypertension		persistently high arterial blood pressure

Glossary		
Word	**Phonetic Prounciation**	**Definition**
induration		the quality of being hard; the process of hardening
ischemic necrosis	(ĭs-kē′mĭk nĕ-krō′sĭs)	death of tissues due to a deficiency of blood
lymphadenopathy	(lĭm-făd″ah-nŏp′ah-thē)	disease of the lymph nodes
MCV		abbreviation for *m*ean *c*orpuscular *v*olume (part of the CBC)
necrotic center	(nĕ-krŏt′ĭk)	death of tissues affecting the central portion of a body part
normocephalic	(nōr″mō-sĕ-făl′ĭk)	pertaining to a normal-appearing head
plts		abbreviation for platelets (formed, noncellular bodies that help coagulate blood)
primary care provider		the physician in charge of your medical records, often seen and dictated as PCP
tetracycline	(tĕt-ră-sī′klēn)	a generic antibiotic
WBCs		abbreviation for *w*hite *b*lood *c*ells

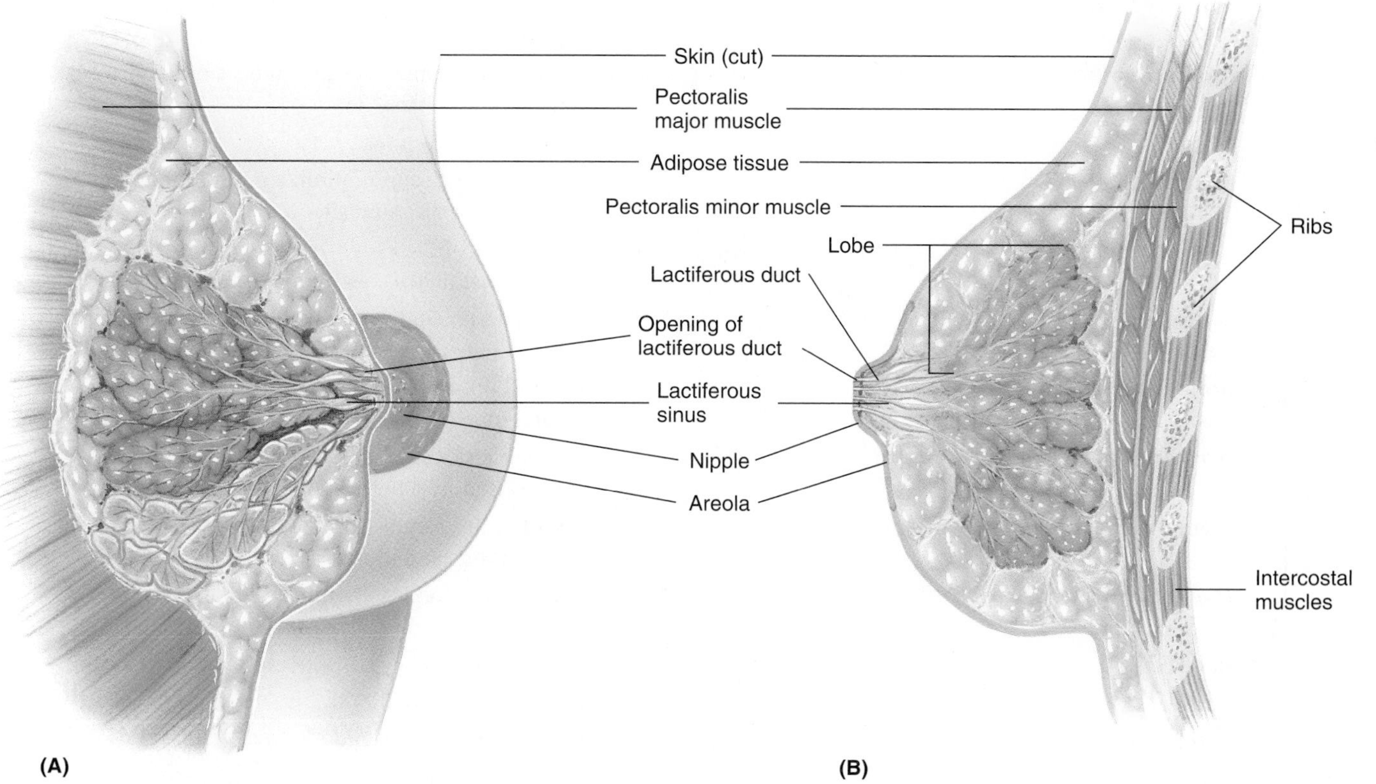
Skin (cut)
Pectoralis major muscle
Adipose tissue
Pectoralis minor muscle
Lobe
Ribs
Lactiferous duct
Opening of lactiferous duct
Lactiferous sinus
Nipple
Areola
Intercostal muscles
(A)
(B)

Figure QC4-1 The Mammary Glands, (A) Anterior View and (B) Sagittal View

REPORT 5: INFECTIOUS DISEASE SOAP NOTE

Jimmy McGann was suffering with cough and congestion, so he went to see his Infectious Disease physician. An AIDS patient, Mr. McGann has been noncompliant with his medications. He received a complete exam with laboratory testing, and medication was prescribed. The patient is to return in a couple of weeks to discuss future therapy. See Figure QC5-1, The Body's Defense Mechanisms, on page 124.

GLOSSARY		
Word	**Phonetic Prounciation**	**Definition**
acute	(ah-kūt′)	having a short and relatively severe course, as in an illness
adenopathy	(ăd″ĕ-nŏp′ah-thē)	enlargement of glands
AIDS		abbreviation for *a*cquired *i*mmuno*d*eficiency *s*yndrome
bronchitis	(brŏng-kī′tĭs)	inflammation of the bronchial tubes
CD4 count		laboratory test to check for the number of CD4 cells (part of the immune system)
CMV hepatitis	(hĕp″ah-tī′tĭs)	inflammation of the liver caused by *c*yto*m*egalo*v*irus (CMV), a herpesvirus
compliance		refers to the patient's following through with his or her established therapeutic plan
cytomegalovirus hepatitis	(sī-tō″mĕg′ah-lō-vī″rŭs)	inflammation of the liver caused by cytomegalovirus, a herpesvirus
diminished breath sounds		when listening to the chest, sounds of breathing are lessened due to illness
GU		abbreviation for *genitourinary*
guarding		a spasm of muscles to minimize motion or agitation of an injured or diseased site
herpes esophagitis	(hĕr′pēz ē-sŏf″ah-jī′tĭs)	inflammation of the esophagus (tube connecting the throat to the stomach) due to a herpesvirus
murmurs		periodic heart sounds; may be heard when listening to the chest
nonproductive cough		cough without expectoration of material from the bronchial tubes
perirectal herpes	(per″ē-rĕk′tăl)	an inflammatory skin disease located around the rectum caused by a herpesvirus
pleuritic chest pain	(plŏo-rĭt′ĭk)	pain within the pleura, which is the serous membrane lining the lungs and thoracic cavity
***Pneumocystis carinii* pneumonia**	(nū-mō-sĭs′tĭs kă-rī′nē-ī)	bacterial pneumonia sometimes seen in AIDS patients
p.o. [L.]		*per os* (by mouth)
p.r.n. [L.]		*pro re nata* (as needed)
q. 6 h. [L.]		every six hours (q.h. stands for *quaque hora*)
range of motion		refers to measuring by the degrees of a circle, the range in which a joint can bend (sometimes dictated "ROM")
rebound (tenderness)		tenderness occurring on release of pressure over an inflamed area of peritoneum
rubs		scraping or grating noises heard with the heartbeat

GLOSSARY

Word	Phonetic Prounciation	Definition
S_1, S_2 *or* S1, S2		first and second heart sounds (normally heard on cardiac exam)
supple		capable of being bent or folded without creases, cracks, or breaks; flexible
Vicodin-Tuss	(vī′kō-dĭn tŭs)	trade name for a medication used as a cough suppressant
viral load		measurement of the amount of virus in a patient, specifically an AIDS patient
Zithromax	(zĭth′rō-măx)	trade name for preparations of azithromycin, an antibiotic
Z-Pak		Zithromax pack containing six capsules of 250 mg each, trade name

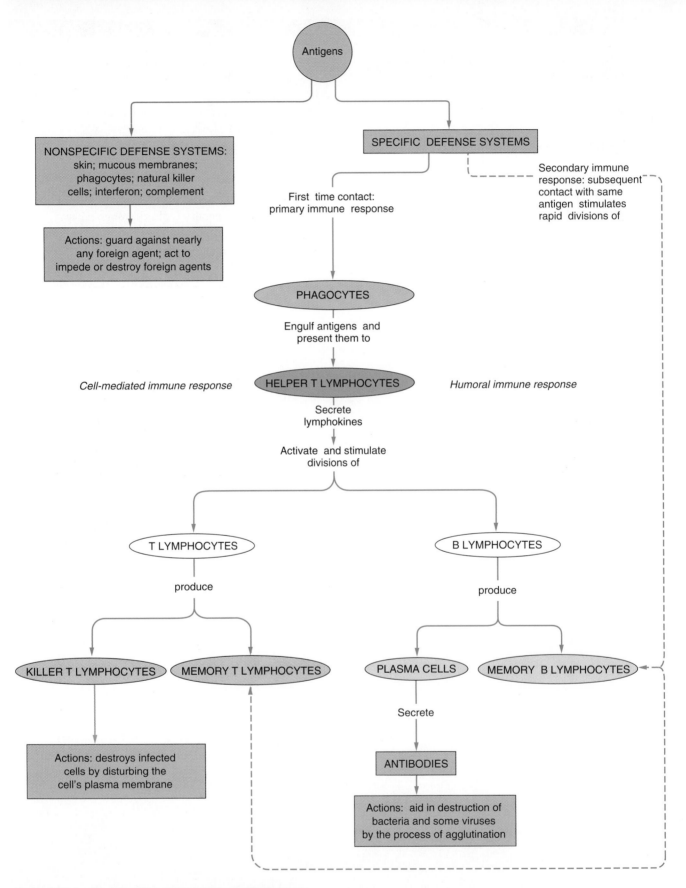

Figure QC5-1   Overview of the Body's Defense Mechanisms

REPORT 6: PULMONOLOGY PROCEDURE NOTE

Doug Peters presented to the Quali-Care Clinic for thoracentesis, a surgical procedure done in the doctor's office.

The procedure was completed without complication, and the patient was advised to return with chest x-rays for further evaluation. A copy of the report was sent to his primary care physician. See Figure QC6-1, Bronchi and Lungs, on page 126.

	GLOSSARY	
Word	**Phonetic Prounciation**	**Definition**
18-gauge Angiocath	(ăn′gē-ō-kăth″)	the size (width) of a specific catheter (trade name) designed to be threaded through an artery
21-gauge needle		the size (width) of a needle
anesthetize	(ah-nĕs′thĕ-tīz)	to put under the influence of anesthetics; drugs or agents used to eliminate the sensation of pain
chest films		x-ray films of the thoracic (chest) area
dyspnea	(dĭsp′nē-ah)	difficult or labored breathing
lateral		pertaining to a side
lidocaine	(lī′dō-kān)	a drug, a local anesthetic, applied to skin and mucous membranes
loculations	(lŏk′ū-lā-shŭnz)	divided into loculi (cavities); sing. loculus
metastatic renal cell carcinoma	(mĕt″ah-stăt′ĭk)	malignancy of kidney cells in which the malignancy has spread to the kidney from another malignant part of the body
PA		abbreviation for *posteroanterior* (from back to front)
pleural effusion	(ploor′ăl ĕ-fū′zhŭn)	the escape of fluid into the pleura (the serous membrane investing the lungs and lining the thoracic cavity)
pleural peel		to remove the outer covering or lining of the pleural cavity
pleurodesis	(ploo-rō-dē′sĭs)	the production of adhesions between the parietal and the visceral pleura
posterolateral thorax	(pō″stĕro-lăt′ĕr-ăl thōr′ăks)	pertaining to the back and side of the thorax (chest)
straw-colored pleural fluid		fluid removed from the thoracic cavity that is described as having the color of straw
therapeutic		pertaining to the treatment of a disease (therapy)
thoracentesis	(thōr″ah-sĕn-tē′sĭs)	surgical puncture of the chest wall for the purpose of draining fluid
ultrasound		a diagnostic technique that uses high-frequency, inaudible sound waves that create a recording (sonogram or echogram) of internal organs

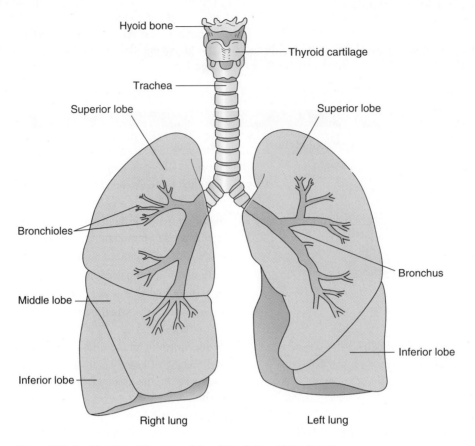

Figure QC6-1   The Branching Bronchi and the Lobes of the Lungs

REPORT 7: ONCOLOGY CONSULT

Jana Stevens has multiple sclerosis. She has been referred to oncology for consultation and possible treatment with mitoxantrone, which may help her spasticity. The patient was given a complete exam, and treatment was begun. Copy of the consult was sent to the requesting physician. See Figure QC7-1, Cranial Nerves, on page 129.

	GLOSSARY	
Word	**Phonetic Prounciation**	**Definition**
Adderall	(ăd′ĕr-ăl)	trade name for an amphetamine used in the treatment of abnormal behavioral syndrome, attention-deficit hyperactivity disorder, and in other abnormalities
affect (n)		physical expression of a person's emotional self
anorexia	(ăn″ō-rĕk′sē-ah)	condition of loss of appetite for food
anxiety		emotional fear or dread of a situation (real or imagined) accompanied by distressful physical symptoms
arthralgia	(ăr-thrăl′jē-ah)	pain in a joint
b.i.d. [L.]		*bis in die* (twice a day)
cardiomyopathy	(kăr′dē-ō-mī-ŏp′-ă-thē)	a general diagnostic term designating primary noninflammatory disease of the heart muscle
conjunctivae	(kŏn-jŭnk-tī′vē)	mucous membrane lining the eyelids and anterior portion of the eyeballs (sing. conjunctiva)
cranial nerves		nerves that carry impulses between the brain, head, and neck regions
D&C		abbreviation for *d*ilation and *c*urettage; stretching of the cervix with various metal dilators and scraping the uterine lining with an instrument called a curette
deep tendon reflexes		involuntary contractions of muscle after a short stretch, caused by percussion of its tendons. This can include the biceps, triceps, and quadriceps reflexes, and others (often seen and dictated as DTRs).
dyspepsia	(dĭs-pĕp′sē-ah)	impairment in the power or function of digestion
epistaxis	(ĕp′ĭ-stăk′sĭs)	nosebleed
EtOH		stands for ethanol, ethyl alcohol
four quadrants		all four quarters of the abdomen
funduscopic (examination)	(fŭn′dŭs-skŏp-ĭk)	pertaining to examining the ocular fundus with an ophthalmoscope
gait incoordination		no purposeful movements
gravida 4, para 1, abortus 3	(grăv′ĭ-dah, păr′ah, ă-bōr′tŭs)	having had four pregnancies with one living child and three miscarriages or abortions
hematochezia	(hē măt ō-kē′zē-ah)	the passage of bloody stools
hematuria	(hēm″ah-tū′rē-ah)	blood in the urine
hemoptysis	(hē-mŏp′tĭ-sĭs)	spitting of blood
L&W		abbreviation for *l*iving and *w*ell
LE		abbreviation for *l*ower *e*xtremity
lymph node	(lĭmf nōd)	a small mass of tissue in the lymphatic system
melena	(mĕl′ĕ-nă)	the passage of black stools; may indicate gastrointestinal hemorrhage

GLOSSARY

Word	Phonetic Prounciation	Definition
miscarriage		a spontaneous abortion of the fetus
mitoxantrone	(mī-tō-zăn′trōn)	generic term for Novantrone
multiple sclerosis		a progressively degenerative neurological disease affecting all aspects of the body
nares patent	(nărēz pā′těnt)	nostrils are open, free of congestion (sing. naris)
neuralgic pain	(nū-răl′jīk)	pertaining to the pain of neuralgia, which exists along the length of one or more nerves
NKDA		abbreviation for *n*o *k*nown *d*rug *a*llergies
Novantrone	(nō-văn′trōn)	trade name for mitoxantrone, a drug used in chemotherapy and to slow the progress of disease in some multiple sclerosis patients
oropharynx	(ō″rō-făr′ĭngks)	division of the pharynx (throat) that lies between the soft palate and the upper edge of the epiglottis
orthopnea	(ŏr″thŏp-nē′ah)	difficult breathing except in an upright position or while using several pillows; may be dictated as three-pillow orthopnea, for example
palpation	(păl-pā′shŭn)	examination by touch
palpitations	(păl″pĭ-tā′shŭnz)	sensation of unduly rapid or irregular heartbeat (should be used in the plural, even if dictated in the singular)
pancytopenia	(păn′sī-tō-pē′nē-ah)	abnormal reduction in erythrocytes, leukocytes, and thrombocytes
pathologic reflexes		reflexes that indicate a disease condition (pathology)
percussion		the act of striking a part with short, sharp blows as an aid in diagnosing the condition of the underlying parts by the sound obtained
PERRLA/EOMI		*p*upils *e*qual, *r*ound, *r*eactive to *l*ight and *a*ccommodation/*e*xtra*o*cular *m*uscles (or movements) *i*ntact (may be separated by a comma or a period)
PMI		*p*oint of *m*aximal *i*mpulse (cardiac term)
PND		*p*aroxysmal *n*octurnal *d*yspnea
polydipsia	(pŏl-ē-dĭp′sē-ah)	excessive thirst for prolonged periods of time
polyuria	(pŏl-ē-yū′rē-ah)	excessive urination for prolonged periods of time
quadriplegic		paralysis in all four extremities
remission		lessening or termination of symptoms of a disease
rigors		stiffness; rigidity
ROS		abbreviation for *r*eview *o*f *s*ystems (a subjective exam)
secondary progressive disease		disease that happens secondary to the progression of a primary disease
self-catheterization	(sělf-kăth′ě-těr-ī-zā′shŭn)	a patient being able to insert a catheter by oneself, maybe at home, with no assistance from health care personnel
SMA		abbreviation for *s*equential *m*ultiple *a*nalyzer; a machine for automated chemical analysis of blood or serum
spasticity	(spas-tĭs′ĭte)	a state or condition of contracted muscles (spasms)

GLOSSARY		
Word	Phonetic Prounciation	Definition
steroids		adrenocortical steroid
tinnitus	(tĭ-nī′tŭs), (tin′ nĭ tŭs)	abnormal noises (ringing) in the ear
TM		abbreviation for *tympanic membrane(s)*
urinary retention		retaining urine
vertigo	(vĕr′tĭ-gō)	dizziness
visceromegaly	(vĭs′ĕr-ō-mĕg′ă-lē)	enlargement of internal organs
vitals stable		phrase that indicates the vital signs (blood pressure, respirations, temperature, pulse rate) are within normal limits
waxed and waned		refers to the increase and subsequent diminishing of an object or symptoms; for example, as the moon waxes and wanes every month, so may symptoms wax and wane or come and go

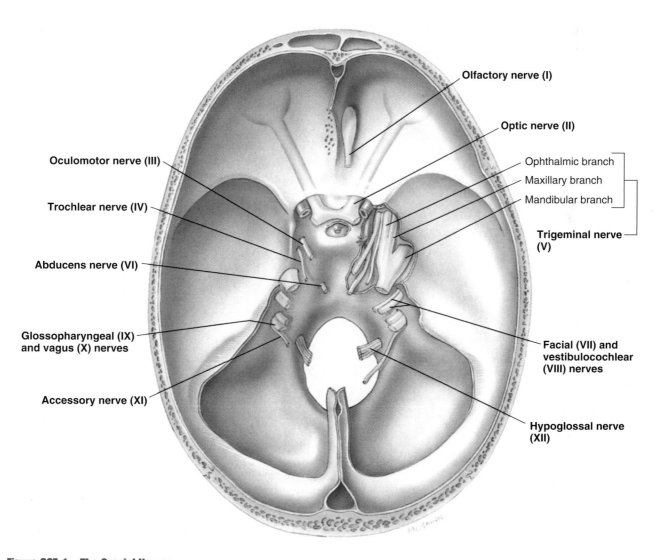

Figure QC7-1 The Cranial Nerves

REPORT 8: CORRESPONDENCE

Her oncology consultant sends a letter to Ms. Stevens's primary care physician, the requesting doctor. The results of her exam and her treatment plan are described. A copy of the letter was forwarded to the psychiatrist to whom the patient has been referred. See Figure QC8-1, Structures of a Neuron.

GLOSSARY		
Word	**Phonetic Prounciation**	**Definition**
marche à petits pas [Fr.]	(mărsh ah pě-tē′pah′)	abnormal gait, taking very short steps
segmental demyelination	(dē-mī′ě-lĭ-nā′shŭn)	degeneration of the myelin sheath of a nerve (or nerves) in segments

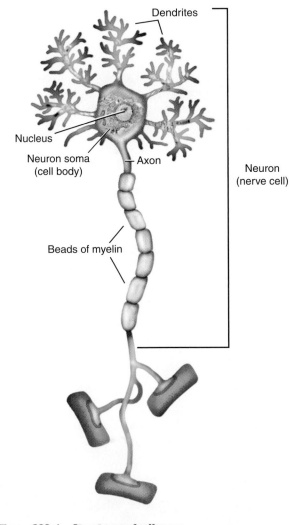

Figure QC8-1   Structures of a Neuron

REPORT 9: INFECTIOUS DISEASE CONSULT

Jorge Romero has been referred by Family Practice to Infectious Disease for a consult due to a long-standing lung lesion. The consulting physician diagnosed the patient's problem, started him on treatment, and scheduled a followup appointment. Copies of the report were sent to the requesting physician, the pulmonologist, and the thoracic surgeon. See Figure QC9-1, Fiberoptic Bronchoscopy, on page 132.

GLOSSARY		
Word	**Phonetic Prounciation**	**Definition**
acid-fast bacilli	(bă-sĭl′ī)	bacilli are rod-shaped bacteria (sing. bacillus); acid-fast refers to a microbiology staining procedure
asymptomatic	(ā′sĭmp-tō-măt′ĭk)	showing or causing no symptoms
bone marrow aspiration and biopsy		removal (aspiration) of bone marrow via needle for diagnostic exam; also, a biopsy of the bone for pathologic exam
bone spur		a small projection from a bone
bronchoscopy	(brŏng-kŏs′kō-pē)	examination of the bronchi via bronchoscope, an instrument used in examination of the tracheobronchial tree
caseating granuloma	(kā-sē-ā′tĭng grăn-ū-lō-mah)	a small group of nodular, inflammatory cells (granuloma) that are soft, dry, crumbling; having a cheesy, necrotic appearance
CNS involvement		abbreviation for *central nervous system* involvement
coccidioidomycosis	(kŏk-sĭd-ē-oy′dō-mī-kō′sĭs)	a fungal disease due to *Coccidioides immitis*
disseminated disease		a disease widely spread throughout either tissue, an organ, or the entire body
erythema	(ĕr″ĭ-thē′mah)	redness of the skin produced by congestion of the capillaries
ethanol		ethyl alcohol
fluconazole	(floo-kŏn′ă-zōl)	generic name for an antifungal agent used either orally or intravenously
fluctuance		the act of moving in waves; to vary in reference to either quantity or quality
fungus		a general term denoting various forms of yeasts and molds
interstitial	(ĭn-tĕr-stĭsh′ăl)	pertaining to spaces within an organ or tissue
joint effusions		escape of fluid from a joint
liver functions		refers to liver function test results
motor 5/5		refers to the function of the motor system (muscles and nerves that produce movement) 5/5 (dictated "five out of five") or normal motor function
needle aspiration		removal of tissue or fluid via needle
non-Hodgkin lymphoma	(lĭm-fō′mah)	malignant tumor of the lymph system *without* the giant Reed-Sternberg cells of Hodgkin disease
organisms		refers to any individual living thing, plant or animal
pulmonary cocci	(kŏk′sī)	bacteria in the lungs (sing. coccus)
pulmonary coccidioidomycosis		a fungal disease in the pulmonary (respiratory) system due to *Coccidioides immitis*

Word	Phonetic Prounciation	Definition
resect		to excise or cut off
sputum		fluid material produced by coughing
titer is >1:8	(tī′tĕr)	a measurement; > means greater than; 1:8 is dictated "one to eight"; titer refers to a substance that has produced a reaction with another substance
toxicity	(tŏk-sĭs′ĭ-tē)	referring to being poisonous
urine cultures		testing urine in a microbiology lab; a sample of urine is placed in a Petri dish—if it is normal, no growth will occur; if abnormal, bacteria will grow over time
washings and cultures		refers to testing fluid obtained from the body (washings) via culture study

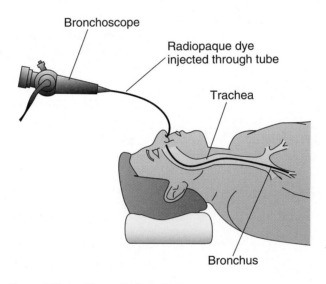

Bronchoscope

Radiopaque dye injected through tube

Trachea

Bronchus

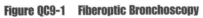

Figure QC9-1   Fiberoptic Bronchoscopy

REPORT 10: PEDIATRICS— EMERGENCY CENTER REPORT

His parents brought Carlos Ledesma to the Quali-Care emergency center with vomiting and headache that had been going on for 24 hours. After evaluation and testing, the boy was diagnosed with viral meningitis and referred to Family Practice for further care. A copy of the report was sent to his family doctor. See Figure QC10-1, Meninges, on page 134.

GLOSSARY		
Word	**Phonetic Prounciation**	**Definition**
0815 hours		military time, which is according to a 24-hour clock; this means 8:15 a.m.
Advil	(ăd′vĭl)	trade name for a nonsteroidal anti-inflammatory drug (ibuprofen)
bacterial process		disease process due to bacterial infection
BP		abbreviation for *b*lood *p*ressure (one of the vital signs)
BRAT diet	(brăt)	abbreviation for *b*ananas, *r*ice *c*ereal, *a*pplesauce, and *t*oast diet
CCP		abbreviation for *c*omplement *c*ontrol *p*rotein
CIE		abbreviation for *c*ounter *i*mmuno*e*lectrophoresis, a test for specific bacterial antigens
CSF		abbreviation for *c*erebro*s*pinal *f*luid
CT brain		abbreviation for *c*omputed *t*omography (x-ray) of the brain
D5$\frac{1}{2}$		abbreviation for a *d*extrose (sugar) and water solution given intravenously
diffuse headache		pain spread throughout the head, not localized to a specific area of the head
fentanyl	(fĕn′tă-nĭl)	generic name for a general anesthetic given intravenously
Gram stain	(grăm)	a method of staining bacteria to look for differences (microscopically) within the bacteria
IV normal saline		a standard saline (salty) solution administered intravenously
L5-S1		pertaining to the vertebral (spinal) column; denoting the fifth lumbar vertebra and the first sacral vertebra
LP		abbreviation for *l*umbar *p*uncture
lymphs	(lĭmfs)	medical jargon; short for lymphocytes, which are white blood cells found in blood or lymph; a part of the white blood cell differential count
meningismus signs	(mĕn″ĭn-jĭs′mŭs)	signs and symptoms of irritation of the meninges due to a high fever or dehydration; no actual infection of the meninges
monos		medical jargon; short for monocytes, a part of the white blood cell differential count
P		abbreviation for *p*ulse (one of the vital signs)

GLOSSARY		
Word	Phonetic Prounciation	Definition
PE tubes		abbreviation for *poly*ethylene *t*ubes, placed in the ears via surgery as treatment for chronic ear infections
Phenergan	(fĕn′ĕr-găn)	trade name for a drug used orally to control nausea and vomiting
Phenergan suppositories		trade name for rectal suppositories used to control nausea and vomiting
polys		medical jargon; short for polymorphonuclear cells, a part of the white blood cell differential count
R		abbreviation for *r*espirations (one of the vital signs)
T		abbreviation for *t*emperature (one of the vital signs)
tonsillectomy	(tŏn′sĭ-lĕk′tō-mē)	surgical removal of the tonsil or tonsils
viral meningitis	(vī′răl mĕn-ĭn-jī′tĭs)	inflammation of the membranes of the brain and/or spinal cord due to a viral infection

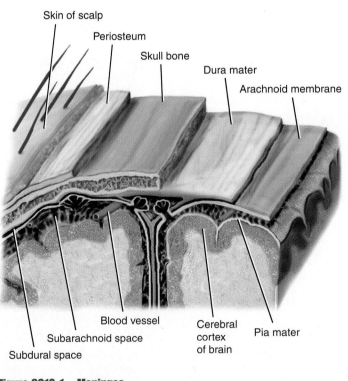

Figure QC10-1   Meninges

REPORT 11: INTERNAL MEDICINE HISTORY AND PHYSICAL

Harold Rivers presented to Internal Medicine for medical clearance before undergoing a neurologic procedure. His-tory and physical exam were completed, and the patient was cleared for the procedure. A copy of the report was sent to the patient's neurologist. See Figures QC11-1, External View of the Eye, and QC11-2, Parts of the Blood, on page 136.

GLOSSARY		
Word	**Phonetic Prounciation**	**Definition**
A&O x3		medical jargon for *a*lert and *o*riented as to person, place, and time; acceptable for use in medical transcription
azotemia	(ăz-ō-tē′mē-ah)	presence of nitrogenous compounds in the blood due to malfunctioning kidneys
bruit [Fr.]	(brwē) (bro͞ot)	a sound or murmur heard on auscultation, especially an abnormal one; primarily used in the plural, bruits
buccal mucosa	(bŭk′ăl mū-kō′săh)	mucous membrane lining the inside of the cheek
DTRs		abbreviation for *d*eep *t*endon *r*eflexes
hyperlipidemia	(hī″pĕr-lĭp″ĭ-dē′mē-ah)	increased concentration of lipids (fatlike substances) in the plasma
idiosyncrasy	(ĭd′ē-ō-sĭn′kră-sē)	a reaction to an agent (food or drug) that is characteristic of an individual
JVD		abbreviation for *j*ugular *v*enous *d*istention (enlarged neck veins)
medical clearance		medical testing or exams designed to clear a patient for a proposed medical procedure
microcytosis	(mī′krō-sī-tō′sĭs)	blood condition in which the erythrocytes are abnormally small
migraine	(mī′grān)	a disorder characterized by recurrent, severe headaches that can be accompanied by nausea and vomiting
neurologic	(nū′rō-lŏj′ĭk)	pertaining to the study of nerves
S₁, S₂, S₃, S₄ *or* S1, S2, S3, S4		first, second, third, and fourth heart sounds; may be heard while listening to the heart via stethoscope; S1 and S2 are normally heard, S3 and S4 are not normally heard
satiety	(sĕ-tī′ĕ-tē)	the state of being fulfilled or satisfied; satiated
sclerae anicteric	(sklēr′ē ăn″ĭk-tĕr′ĭk)	no jaundice of the sclerae (outer white layer of the eyes)
spondylolisthesis	(spŏn′dĭ-lō-lĭs-thē′sĭs)	an abnormal condition in which one vertebra has a forward displacement over another vertebra, due either to a fracture or a congenital defect
vascular headache		pain in the head due to abnormal dilatation of meningeal arteries
Zocor	(zō′kōr)	a preparation of simvastatin, a medication used to lower the level of lipids (fats) in the blood (trade name)

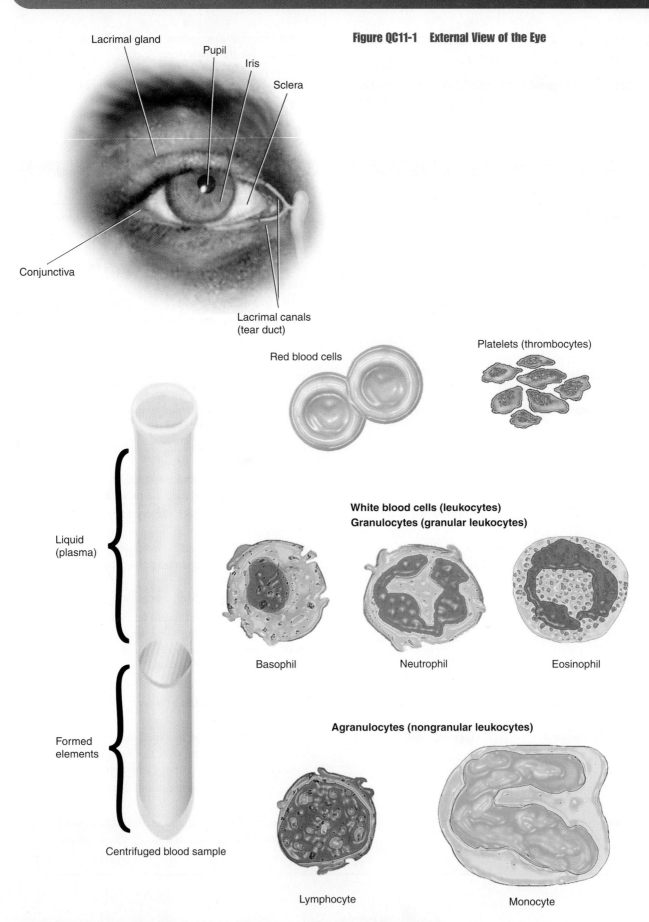

Lacrimal gland

Pupil

Iris

Sclera

Figure QC11-1   External View of the Eye

Conjunctiva

Lacrimal canals
(tear duct)

Red blood cells

Platelets (thrombocytes)

Liquid
(plasma)

White blood cells (leukocytes)
Granulocytes (granular leukocytes)

Basophil

Neutrophil

Eosinophil

Formed
elements

Agranulocytes (nongranular leukocytes)

Centrifuged blood sample

Lymphocyte

Monocyte

Figure QC11-2   Plasma, Formed Elements, Erythrocytes, Leukocytes, and Thrombocytes

REPORT 12: PSYCHIATRY CONSULT

Barbara Ann Richards is a young woman who was referred
to Psychiatry because of a bad experience with drug abuse.
She also has had suicidal tendencies.

GLOSSARY		
Word	**Phonetic Prounciation**	**Definition**
chemotherapy	(kē″mō-thār′-ă-pē)	treatment of disease by chemical agents
EMS		*E*mergency *M*edical *S*ervices
GAF scale		*G*lobal *A*ssessment of *F*unction scale (from 1 to 100) used in studies of treatment effectiveness
psychotherapy	(sī-kō-thār′ă-pē)	treatment of mental disorders and behavioral disturbances

REPORT 13: RADIOLOGY—ECHOCARDIOGRAM REPORT

Maggie Ricks underwent a preoperative echocardiogram, the results of which subsequently proved acceptable for the patient to go forward with her planned gastrointestinal surgical procedure. Copies of the x-ray test results were sent to her GI physician and to her general surgeon. See Figures QC13-1, Echocardiograph below and QC13-2, Cardiac Cycle and ECG Reading, on page 139.

GLOSSARY		
Word	Phonetic Prounciation	Definition
aortic valve	(ā-ōr′tĭk)	a valve that regulates blood flow between the left ventricle and the aorta
color flow study		color images via ultrasound; a radiologic procedure
Doppler	(Dŏp′lĕr)	instrument named for Christian Doppler; used in ultrasonography, a radiologic procedure (Doppler color flow imaging)
echocardiogram	(ĕk-ō-kăr′dē-ō-grăm)	an image produced by echocardiography (exam of the heart by ultrasound)
ejection fraction		that fraction of the volume of blood in the ventricles of the heart at the end of diastole (dilatation) that is expelled during systole (contraction)
inflow pattern		pattern of blood flow as it enters the vessels of the heart
mitral valve	(mī′trăl)	the valve that regulates blood flow between the left atrium and the left ventricle of the heart
peak aortic valve velocity		the maximum rate of movement of the aortic valve
pericardial effusion	(per-ĭ-kăr′dē-ăl ĕ-fū′zhŭn)	escape of fluid into the pericardium (area around the heart)
systolic pulmonary artery pressure	(sĭs-tŏl′ĭk pŭl′mō-nār-ē)	pressure in the pulmonary artery during systole
mitral regurgitation		backflow of blood from the left atrium into the left ventricle of the heart
trivial		of little importance
ventricular thrombus	(vĕn-trĭk′ū-lăr thrŏm′bŭs)	a blood clot in a ventricle

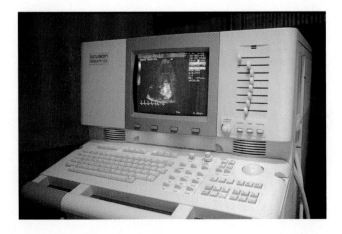

Figure QC13-1　Echocardiograph (Photo by Marcia Butterfield. Courtesy of W.A. Foote Memorial Hospital, Jackson, MI)

Q wave is a negative deflection or wave.

R wave is a positive deflection or wave.

S wave is a negative wave.

T wave is a positive wave and represents ventricular repolarization.

U wave (occasionally seen in some patients) is a positive deflection and associated with repolarization.

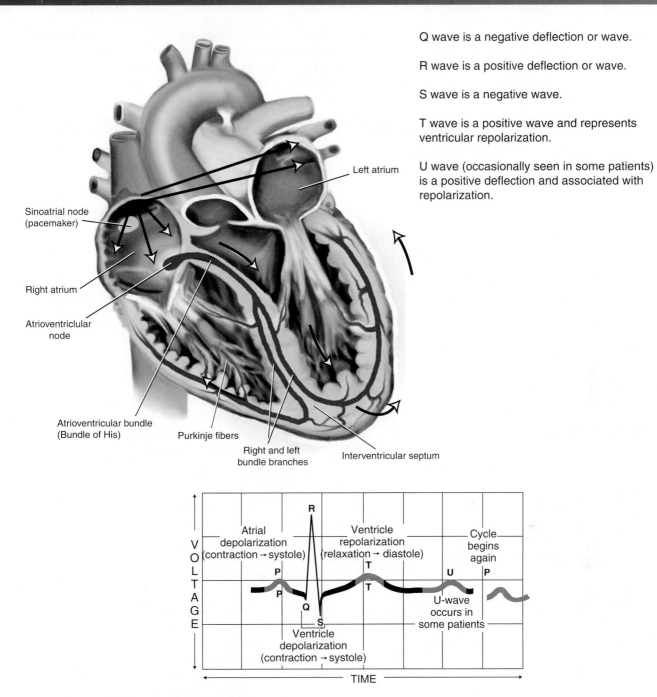

Figure QC13-2   Cardiac Cycle and ECG Reading

REPORT 14: RADIOLOGY— COLONOSCOPY PROCEDURE NOTE

Leon Markowitz, a patient with multiple medical problems, required a colonoscopy prior to his scheduled heart surgery. The procedure was done in his gastroenterologist's clinic with copies of the findings sent to the patient's cardiac surgeon and to his hematologist. See Figures QC14-1, The Large Intestine, and QC14-2, Colonoscope, on page 141.

	GLOSSARY	
Word	Phonetic Prounciation	Definition
ICD code 211.3		*I*nternational *C*lassification of *D*iseases: A standard list of identifying codes used in statistics, billing, etc.; the code 211.3 relates to a benign neoplasm of the colon
ICD code 562.10		relates to diverticulitis of the colon
anticoagulated	(ăn′tē-kō-ăg′ū-lāt-ĕd)	treated with a substance added to prevent coagulation (blood clots)
ascending colon	(ă-sĕnd′ĭng kō′lŏn)	a section of the large intestine that connects the cecum to the transverse colon
cecum	(sē′kŭm)	the first section of the large intestine
colonoscopy	(kō-lŏn-ŏs′kŏ-pē)	visual examination of the colon by means of an endoscope
coronary artery bypass surgery	(kōr′ŏ-nār-ē)	a section of vein surgically grafted between the aorta and a coronary artery in order to bypass an obstruction in the artery
descending colon	(dē-sĕnd′ĭng)	a section of the large intestine connecting the transverse colon to the sigmoid colon
diverticula	(dī-vĕr-tĭk′ū-lă)	abnormal pouches or sacs in the intestinal wall (sing. diverticulum)
excisional biopsies		tissues removed at surgery for microscopic examination
iron deficiency anemia		blood condition deficient in iron
myocardial infarction	(mī″ō-kăr′dē-ăl ĭn-fărk′shŭn)	gross necrosis of the myocardium as a result of interruption of the blood supply to the heart (heart attack)
peptic ulcer disease	(pĕp′tĭk)	pathologic condition that causes ulceration of the esophagus, stomach, and/or duodenum
sessile polyp	(sĕs īl′ pŏl′ĭp)	stemlike connected growth or mass protruding from a mucous membrane
snare	(snār)	surgical instrument used for excising stemlike connected growths by excising them at their base
transverse colon		a section of the large intestine connecting the ascending colon to the descending colon
valve		a membranous fold in a passage or canal to prevent reflux (backward flow) of the substance flowing through it
Versed	(vĕr-sĕd′)	trade name for a nonbarbiturate agent given intravenously either before or during surgery to produce both sedation and amnesia
Xylocaine	(zī′lō-kān)	trade name for an anesthetic drug administered topically

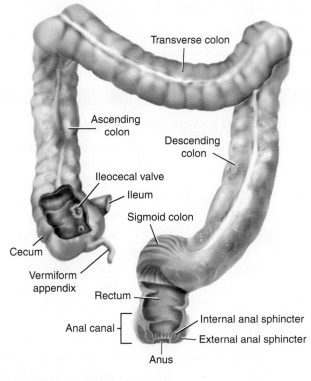
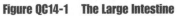

Figure QC14-1 The Large Intestine

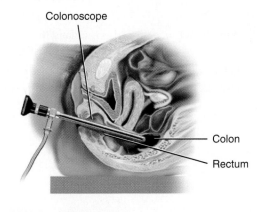

Figure QC14-2 Colonoscopy

REPORT 15: RADIOLOGY—CT SCAN OF ABDOMEN

Maggie Ricks had another preoperative test—a CT scan of her abdomen. The results illustrated her gastrointestinal problems. Copies of these findings were sent to her GI physician and to her general surgeon. See Figure QC15-1, Computed Tomography.

GLOSSARY		
Word	**Phonetic Prounciation**	**Definition**
12 Hounsfield units		units of x-ray attenuation used in CT scans; symbol H
adrenal glands	(ă-drē′năl)	glands that secrete hormones
attenuation	(ă-tĕn-ū-ā′shŭn)	to reduce the energy of a beam of radiation; to lessen the severity of a condition
axial scans	(ăk′sē-ăl)	x-ray images of the axis (meeting point) of two structures
basal atelectatic changes	(bā′săl ăt-ĕ-lĕk-tăt′ĭk)	changes due to the absence of air from air-containing cells (alveoli) at the lung base(s)
basal parenchymal densities	(pă-rĕng′kĭ-măl)	dense areas in the base of the functional elements of an organ
bilateral or bilaterally		pertaining to both sides
coronal fascia	(kōr′ō-năl făsh′ē-ah)	a band of deep tissue with the shape of a horn
costophrenic angle	(kŏs-tō-frĕn′ĭk)	an angle formed on either side of the diaphragm and the ribs
diffusely		not localized but spread throughout
enteric contrast	(ĕn-tĕr′ĭk)	substance introduced into the small intestine to help in defining the radiologic images obtained
hydronephrosis	(hī′drō-nĕ-frō′sĭs)	abnormal condition of fluid within the kidneys
intravenous contrast	(ĭn′tră-vē′nŭs)	contrast medium (dye) inserted through a vein prior to taking an x-ray
lateral		pertaining to a side
pancreas	(păn′krē-ăs)	a gland that secretes digestive juices into the small intestine
perisplenic fluid collection	(pĕr-ĭ-splĕn′ĭk)	collection of fluid around the spleen
subsegmental atelectasis	(ăt-ĕ-lĕk′tă-sĭs)	absence of air or obstruction of an organ in small segments

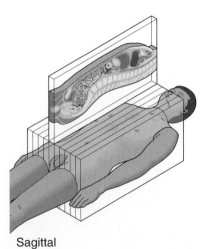
Sagittal

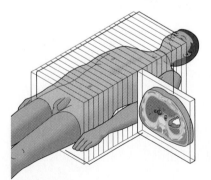
Transverse

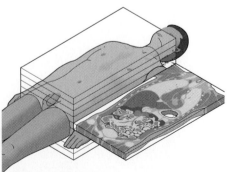
Coronal (frontal)

Figure QC15-1   Computed Tomography

REPORT 16: INFECTIOUS DISEASE HPIP NOTE

Otto Werner Valtin, a known AIDS patient, has been feeling ill. He went to his Internist for an exam. The doctor scheduled the patient for testing and a radiologic procedure. He also referred Mr. Valtin to a dentist. The patient was scheduled to return to Internal Medicine when the results of his tests and x-rays are available. See Figures QC16-1, Thrush, and QC16-2, Structures of a Tooth, on page 144.

	GLOSSARY	
Word	**Phonetic Prounciation**	**Definition**
amylase	(ăm′ě-lās)	an enzyme that helps in the conversion of starch into sugar
BS		abbreviation for *bowel sounds*
caries	(kār′ēz)	tooth decay
crackles		an abnormal rattling sound heard on auscultation of the chest; also referred to as rales
CVA		abbreviation for *cardiovascular accident*
discrete mass		a lump that is clearly distinct from its surroundings
expiratory wheezes	(ĕk-spī′ră-tō-rē)	a whistling sound heard on expiration (breathing out)
MAI		abbreviation for *Mycobacterium avium-intracellulare*
Mycobacterium avium-intracellulare	(mī′kō-băk-tēr′ē-um av′ē-ŭm ĭn′tră-sĕl′ū-lār-ā)	genus and species of bacteria that cause systemic disease in immunocompromised patients, e.g., AIDS patients
oral thrush		disease (lesions) of the mouth, lips, and throat caused by fungus
periodontal disease	(pĕr′ē-ō-dŏn′tăl)	gum disease
ROM		abbreviation for *range of motion*
SOB		abbreviation for *shortness of breath*
straight-leg raise		patient raising the legs, one at a time, straight into the air; part of a neurologic exam
supraclavicular	(sū-pră-klă-vĭk′ū-lăr)	situated or located above the clavicle (collar bone)
viral load		the measurable quantity of virus in a patient's blood stream, especially an AIDS patient

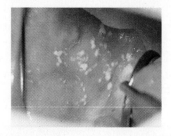

Figure QC16-1   Thrush (Courtesy of Dr. Joseph Konzelman, School of Dentistry, Medical College of Georgia)

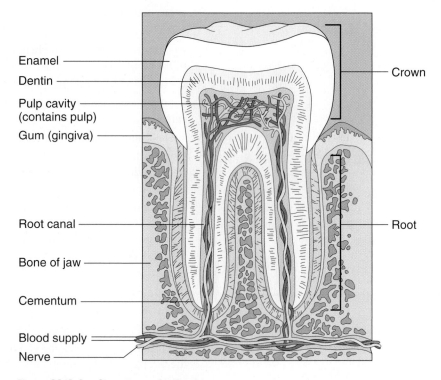

Enamel

Dentin

Pulp cavity
(contains pulp)

Gum (gingiva)

Crown

Root canal

Bone of jaw

Cementum

Blood supply

Nerve

Root

Figure QC16-2   Structures of a Tooth

REPORT 17: RADIOLOGY—MAMMOGRAM AND CT SCAN OF ABDOMEN

Doris Dean had her yearly mammogram today along with CT scans of her abdomen and pelvis. She completed the mammogram and was prepared for her CT scans by being given contrast material, both intravenously and orally. Copies of the results were sent to the referring physician. See Figure QC17-1, Mammography, on page 146.

GLOSSARY		
Word	**Phonetic Prounciation**	**Definition**
aorta	(ā-ōr′tă)	the artery that carries blood out of the heart
axial images	(ăk′sē-ăl)	routine x-ray images taken on the axis, the line around which the body turns
cortex	(kōr′tĕks)	the outer layer of an internal organ
hemipelvis	(hĕm′ē-pĕl′vĭs)	one-half of the pelvis
iliac fossa	(ĭl′ē-ăk fŏs′ah)	a depressed area of the ilium that is the uppermost and largest portion of the pelvis
Isovue-300	(ī′sō-vū)	trade name for preparations of iopamidol (a nonionic radiopaque medium used in x-ray procedures)
IV		abbreviation for *intra*venous
mammogram	(măm′ō-grăm)	a radiograph (x-ray film) of the breast
medial	(mē′dē-ăl)	pertaining to the middle
microcalcifications	(mī′krō-kăl sĭ-fĭ-kā′shŭnz)	minute (small) amounts of calcium salts
nodule	(nŏd′yūl)	a small knot or lump that is harder than the surrounding tissue and is perceptible by touch
oblique view	(ŏb-lēk′)	a slanting positional and/or directional view
omental thickening	(ō-mĕn′tăl)	thickening of the omentum, which is a fold of the peritoneum connecting the stomach and other internal organs
parenchyma	(pă-reng′kĭ-mă)	the functional portion of an organ as opposed to its framework
radiopacities	(rā′dē-ō-păs′ĭ-tēz)	obstruction of radiant energy allowing for white areas on an x-ray film

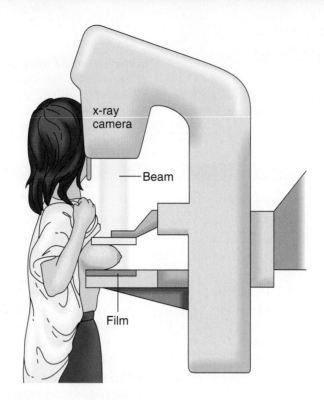

x-ray camera

Beam

Film

Figure QC17-1   Mammography

REPORT 18: ONCOLOGY CONSULT

This elderly gentleman was referred for an oncology consult to rule out metastatic carcinoma. Sterling Peak is a known cancer patient, having undergone a Whipple procedure five years ago. A copy of this consult was sent to Dr. Mooney, Internal Medicine. See Figure QC18-1, the Anatomy of the Pancreas, on page 148.

	GLOSSARY	
Word	**Phonetic Prounciation**	**Definition**
5-FU		abbreviation for 5-*fluorou*racil, an intravenous anticancer drug
A&P		abbreviation for *a*uscultation (listening) and *p*ercussion (feeling)
angina	(ăn-jī′nah) (ăn′jĕ-nah)	spasmodic, choking, or suffocating pain
arthralgias	(ăr-thrăl′-jē-ăs)	pains in joints
Bright disease		broad, descriptive term for a kidney disease
cholestyramine	(kō les tī ră mēn)	medication used in hypercholesterolemia (high levels of cholesterol in the blood)
CPT-11		abbreviation for *Campt*osar, an anticancer drug (generic, irinotecan)
Effexor	(ē′fĕx-ŏr)	trade name for an antidepressant medication (generic, venlafaxine)
empyema	(ĕm-pī-ē′mah)	buildup of pus in a body cavity
gait	(gāt)	method of walking
Gemzar	(jĕm′zăr)	trade name for an anticancer drug (generic, gemcitabine)
genitalia	(jĕn′ĭ-tā′lē-ah)	external reproductive organs
GI		abbreviation for *gastro*i*ntestinal*
Hemoccult	(hē′mō-kŭlt)	trade name for a test to discover occult (hidden) blood in the stool
heterogeneity	(hĕt′ĕr-ō-jĕ-nē′ĭ-tē)	composed of unrelated elements
homogeneous	(hō-mō-jē′nē-ŭs)	composed of similar elements
leucovorin	(lū′kō-vōr-ĭn)	an agent used to treat anemia
Lomotil	(lō mō′tĭl)	trade name for a drug used in the treatment of diarrhea
metastasis	(mĕ-tăs′tă-sĭs)	spread of disease process from one part of the body to another (pl. metastases)
MRI		abbreviation for *m*agnetic *r*esonance *i*maging
MVA		abbreviation for *m*otor *v*ehicle *a*ccident
picograms/mL	(pī′kō-grămz)	a metric unit of mass (weight) per milliliter, abbreviated pg/mL (The virgule is dictated as "per.")
psoriasis	(sō-rī′ă-sĭs)	a skin disease distinguished by scaly, reddish patches
thermal ablation	(thĕrm′ăl ăb-lā′shŭn)	removal or separation of tissue using heat
vertigo	(vĕr′ tĭ-gō)	dizziness
vipoma	(vĭ-pō′mah)	an endocrine tumor, appearing most often in the pancreas
Wellbutrin	(wĕl-bū′trĭn)	trade name for an antidepressant medication (generic, bupropion)
Whipple procedure		radical surgical procedure consisting of excision of the duodenum, the distal third of the stomach, and the head of the pancreas

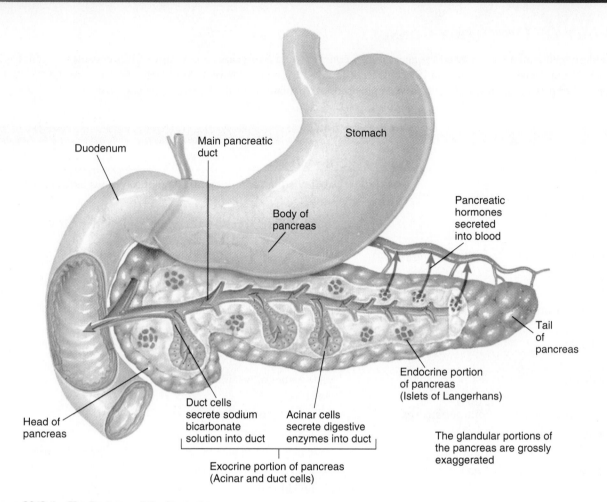

Duodenum

Main pancreatic duct

Stomach

Body of pancreas

Pancreatic hormones secreted into blood

Tail of pancreas

Endocrine portion of pancreas (Islets of Langerhans)

Duct cells secrete sodium bicarbonate solution into duct

Acinar cells secrete digestive enzymes into duct

The glandular portions of the pancreas are grossly exaggerated

Head of pancreas

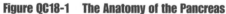

Exocrine portion of pancreas (Acinar and duct cells)

Figure QC18-1   The Anatomy of the Pancreas

REPORT 19: CORRESPONDENCE

Dr. McCracken, oncologist, sent a letter to Sterling Peak's primary care provider (Dr. Jean Mooney) describing his evaluation, findings, and plan for Mr. Peak. See Figure QC19-1, The Anatomy of the Liver.

GLOSSARY		
Word	Phonetic Prounciation	Definition
hepatic resection	(hē-păt′ĭk rē-sĕk′shŭn)	surgical excision of a portion of the liver
Questran	(kwĕs′trăn)	trade name for medication used in hypercholesterolemia

Figure QC19-1   The Anatomy of the Liver

REPORT 20: PULMONOLOGY—SLEEP STUDY

John J. Crawford was experiencing excessive daytime sleepiness and was sent for a sleep study, which involved two separate nights. The first night's study showed severe sleep apnea, but the second night's study was unable to be completed due to the patient's inability to tolerate the mask that was used. He was referred to psychiatry for evaluation and treatment of his claustrophobia. See Figures QC20-1, Larynx, Trachea, and Bronchial Tree, and QC20-2, CPAP Machine, on page 152.

GLOSSARY		
Word	**Phonetic Prounciation**	**Definition**
Altace	(ăl′tās)	an antihypertensive medication (trade name)
anterior tibialis muscle	(ăn-tēr′ē-ĕr tĭb-ē-ŭ′lĭs)	muscle in front of the tibia (shin bone)
apnea	(ăp ′nē-ah)	absence of breathing
Atrovent	(ăt′rō-vĕnt)	a bronchodilator medication (trade name)
BiPAP	(bī′păp)	abbreviation for *bi*level *p*ositive *a*irway *p*ressure
cataplexy	(kăt′ă-plĕk-sē)	physical condition characterized by muscle weakness resulting from a severe emotional state; anger or fear
claustrophobic	(klăw-strō-fō-′bĭk)	a severe emotional state resulting from fear of enclosed spaces
CPAP titration	(sē′păp tī-trā′shŭn)	abbreviation for *c*ontinuous *p*ositive *a*irway *p*ressure, adjustment of
distended		stretched or enlarged
EEG		abbreviation for *electro*encephalogram
electromyogram	(ē-lĕk-trō-mī′ō-grăm)	an x-ray (electrical tracing) of muscle (sometimes dictated EMG)
electro-oculogram	(ē-lĕk′trō-ŏk′ū-lō-grăm)	an x-ray (electrical tracing) of eye movements
EOMI		abbreviation for *extra*ocular *m*ovements (or muscles) intact
gastroesophageal reflux	(găs′trō-ē-sŏf′ă-jē′ăl)	reflux (backward flow) of the digested contents of the stomach into the esophagus
hypnagogic hallucinations	(hĭp-nă-gŏj′ĭk)	hallucinations caused by the onset of sleep
hypopnea	(hī-pŏp′nē-ah)	abnormal decrease in the rate of inspiration and expiration
intercostal	(ĭn-tĕr-kŏs′tŏl)	pertaining to between the ribs
Lasix	(lā′sĭks)	trade name for medication used as a diuretic
leg edema	(ĕ-dē′mah)	swelling (fluid accumulation) in the intercellular tissues of the leg or legs
macroglossia	(măk-rō-glŏs′ē-ah)	condition of enlarged tongue
midline		the division of the body into right and left halves using an imaginary line
night sweats		profuse sweating at nighttime
nocturia	(nŏk-tū′rē-ah)	excessive urination during the nighttime
polysomnogram	(pŏl-ē-sŏm′nō-grăm)	graphic tracing of various physiologic variables recorded during sleep for the detection of physiologic causes of sleep disorders
polysomnography	(pŏl-ē-sŏm-nŏg′ră-fē)	the process of recording a polysomnogram (sleep study)

GLOSSARY		
Word	**Phonetic Prounciation**	**Definition**
precordial EKG lead	(prē-kōr′dē-ăl)	wire connected to the chest wall during an EKG (electrocardiographic tracing of the electrical activity of the heart)
pulse oximeter	(ŏk-sĭm′ĕ-tĕr)	an instrument used to measure oxygen saturation of the blood in a capillary (sometimes dictated pulse ox)
rebound tenderness		tenderness of a part of the body felt upon withdrawal of a stimulus
REM sleep	(rĕm)	abbreviation for a phase of deep sleep defined by *rapid eye movements*
Respitrace unit	(rĕs′pĭ-trās)	machine used in sleep studies to measure airflow from the nose and mouth, trade name
sleep latency	(lā′tĕn-sē)	the time period (onset) of sleep
soft palate	(păl′ăt)	the fleshy formation located at the top (back) of the mouth
summed respiratory movements		total amount of movements made during breathing process
supine	(sū-pīn′)	lying on the back with the face upward
trachea	(trā′kē-ah)	windpipe

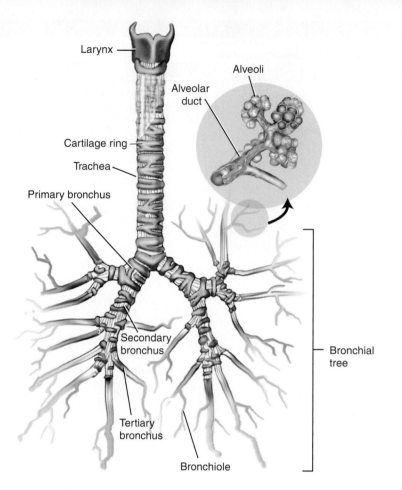

Figure QC20-1   Larynx, Trachea, and Bronchial Tree

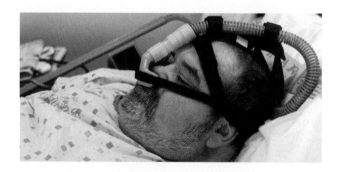

Figure QC20-2   CPAP Machine

REPORT 21: PSYCHIATRY CONSULT

Leslie Arispe is an elderly woman with dementia and depression who is also suicidal. She was referred to Psychiatry for examination and for treatment recommendations.

GLOSSARY		
Word	Phonetic Prounciation	Definition
arcus senilis	(ăr′kŭs sē nīl-ĭs)	opaque white ring about the periphery of the cornea, seen in patients >50 years of age
Ativan	(ăt′ĭ-văn)	lorazepam, an antianxiety drug (trade name)
benzodiazepines	(bĕn′zō-dī-ăz′ĕ-pĕnz)	class of drugs used to treat anxiety and insomnia
bradycardia	(brăd-ē-kăr′dē-ah)	slowness of the heartbeat
cholecystectomy	(kō′lē-sĭs-tĕk′tō-mē)	surgical removal of the gallbladder
dementia	(dē-mĕn′shē-ah)	loss or impairment of intellectual abilities due to organic causes
Depakote	(dĕp′ă-kōt)	divalproex sodium, a drug used to treat seizures (trade name)
dysuria	(dĭs-ū′rē-ah)	painful or difficult urination
EKG, ECG		*e*lectro*c*ardiogram (EKG and ECG are both correct)
flurazepam	(floor-ăz′ĕ-păm)	generic nonbarbiturate drug used for insomnia
Haldol	(hăl′dŏl)	haloperidol, an antipsychotic drug (trade name)
hypercholesterolemia	(hī″pĕr-kō-lĕs″tĕr-ŏl-ē′mē-ah)	excessive levels of cholesterol in the blood
hyperglycemia	(hī″pĕr-glī-sē′mē-ah)	abnormally increased levels of glucose (sugar) in the blood
hypotensive	(hī″pō-tĕn′sĭv)	abnormally low blood pressure
hypovolemia	(hī″pō-vō-lē′mē-ah)	a decreased amount of blood (plasma) in the body
hysterectomy	(hĭs″tĕ-rĕck′tō-mē)	excision of the entire uterus; may be performed either laparoscopically, through an abdominal incision, or vaginally
ketoacidosis	(kē″tō-ăs″ĭ-dō′sĭs)	acidosis together with the buildup of ketone bodies in tissues and fluids
lithium	(lĭth′ē-ŭm)	drug used for manic-depressive disorders
Paxil	(păx′ĭl)	trade name for an antidepressant agent (generic, paroxetine hydrochloride)
Premarin	(prĕm′ăh-rĭn)	trade name for estrogen replacement drug used in menopausal patients
somnolent	(sŏm′nō-lĕnt)	sleepiness; drowsy
trazodone	(trā′zō-dōn, also tră′zō dōn)	an antidepressant drug, generic
urinalysis	(ū″rĭ-năl′ĭ-sĭs)	chemical or microscopic analysis of urine
Vasotec	(văs′ō-tĕk)	an inhibitor drug used for hypertension (generic, enalapril maleate); trade name
verapamil	(vĕr″ăh-păm′ĭl)	generic drug used for angina, arrhythmias, and hypertension; also used for migraine headaches
vulvectomy	(vŭl-vĕk′tō-mē)	excision of the vulva

REPORT 22: RADIOLOGY—MRI

Emily Pickens was sent to radiology for MRI studies because of a questionable area in her right lower extremity found on orthopedic examination. The findings were benign, and copies of the report were sent to her pediatrician and to the orthopedic doctor who had requested the MRI. See Figures QC22-1, to the right, Magnetic Resonance Imaging; QC22-2, on page 155, Superficial Muscles of the Leg; and QC22-3, The Femur, on page 156.

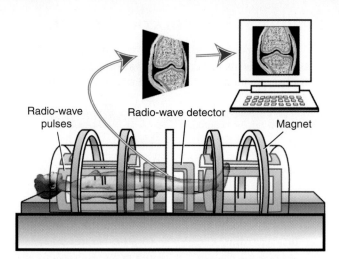

Radio-wave pulses   Radio-wave detector   Magnet

Figure QC22-1   Schematic of Magnetic Resonance Imaging

GLOSSARY		
Word	**Phonetic Prounciation**	**Definition**
82 slices		refers to the number of times the MRI equipment cuts through the tissue, making images (the number can vary)
axial	(ăk′sē-ăl)	an imaginary line depicting the center of the body
expansile	(ĕks-păn′sĭl)	relative to expanding
fascial	(făsh′ē-ăl)	pertaining to the supportive layer of thin, connective tissues (fascia) within the muscles and/or organs of the body
fibrous	(fī′brŭs)	tissue composed of or containing fibers, which are elongated, threadlike structures
fibular epiphysis	(fĭb′ū-lăr ĕ-pĭf′ĭ-sĭs)	the end portion of the fibula, which is the smaller of the two lower leg bones; "growth plate" of the fibula
hematoma	(hēm″ăh-tō′mah)	a mass or collection of blood (plural, hematomata)
hypointense	(hī″pō-ĭn-tĕns′)	pertaining to a low intensity
lateral compartment	(lăt′ĕr-ăl)	pertaining to the side of a small enclosure within a larger space
MRI		*m*agnetic *r*esonance *i*maging
neoplasm	(nē′ō-plăzm)	new growth of tissue; oftentimes relative to a tumor
PDWI		abbreviation for *p*roton *d*ensity-*w*eighted *i*maging (used in MRI)
proximal	(prŏk′sĭ-măl)	nearest; closer to any point of reference
sagittal	(săj′ĭ-tăl)	an imaginary vertical plane that divides the body or any structure pertaining to the body into right and left sides
satellite lesions	(lē′zhŭns)	smaller lesions located near a larger lesion
subcutaneous	(sŭb″kū-tā′nē-ŭs)	pertaining to beneath the skin
T1WI		abbreviation for T1-*w*eighted *i*maging
T2WI		abbreviation for T2-*w*eighted *i*maging

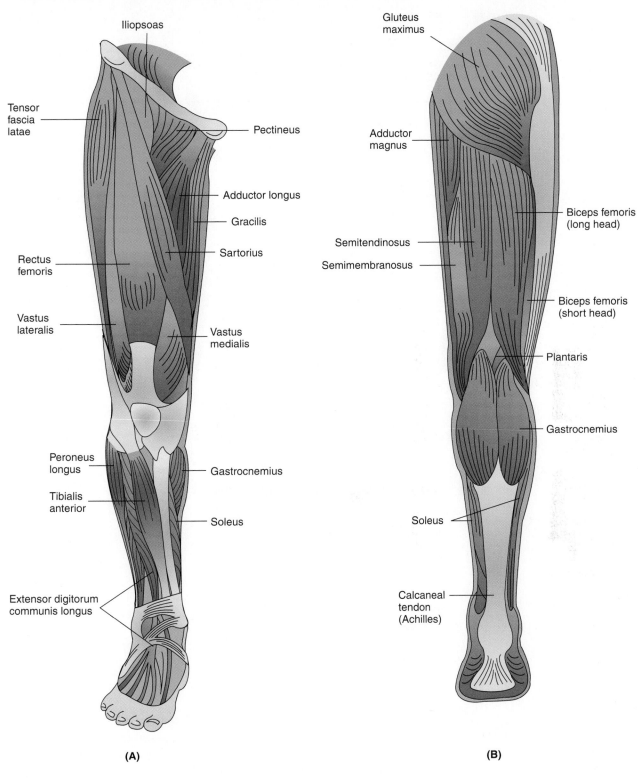

Figure QC22-2 Superficial Muscles of the Leg, (A) Anterior View (B) Posterior View

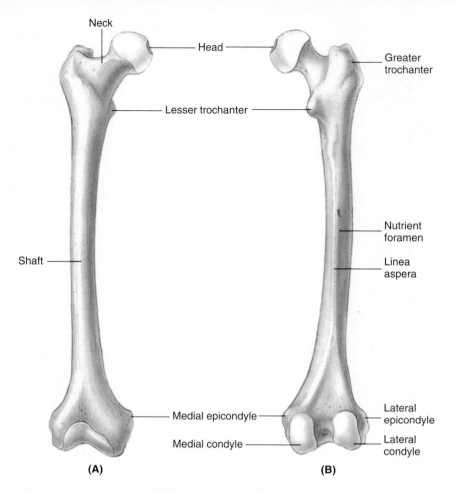

Neck

Head

Greater
trochanter

Lesser trochanter

Nutrient
foramen

Linea
aspera

Shaft

Medial epicondyle

Lateral
epicondyle

Medial condyle

Lateral
condyle

(A)

(B)

Figure QC22-3   The Femur, (A) Anterior View (B) Posterior View

REPORT 23: PEDIATRICS— EMERGENCY CENTER REPORT

Her parents brought B. Christine Anello to the Emergency Center after she had been burned at home by an overturned crockpot. After a complete exam, the ER physician dis-cussed the case with Charles Lanier, MD, intensivist. Christine was transferred to the Hillcrest pediatric intensive care unit under Dr. Lanier's care. A copy of the ER report was sent to her pediatrician, Chris Salem, DO. See Figures QC23-1A, B, and C, Burns, on page 158.

GLOSSARY		
Word	**Phonetic Prounciation**	**Definition**
1700 hours		military time for 5 p.m.
bicarb	(bī′kărb)	abbreviation for bicarbonate, a bodily salt
chloride	(klōr′īd)	a salt consisting of hydrochloric acid
circumferential		the distance measured by a line that is encompassing a circle
electrolytes	(ē-lĕk′trō-līts)	any liquid substance that is capable of conducting an electrical current
extraocular	(ĕks-tră-ŏk′ū-lăr)	pertaining to outside the eye
first- and second-degree burns		lesions that affect the superficial epidermis, the epidermis, and the dermis (various layers of skin) See Lund and Browder burn chart, page 197 in the Appendix.
icterus	(ĭk′tĕr-ŭs)	jaundice; yellowish color of the skin or sclerae
intensivist	(ĭn-tĕn′sĭ-vĭst)	physician specializing in the care of patients in an intensive care unit
Lund Browder chart		a burn extent estimator (see page 197 in the Appendix)
perineum	(pĕr′ĭ-nē′ŭm)	the area of the anatomy located between the thighs extending from the vulva to the anus in a female or from the scrotum to the anus in a male
potassium		chemical element (alkaline salts) that maintains an acid-base and water balance in the body; symbol K
PT		*p*rothrombin *t*ime, a test to determine coagulation, sometimes dictated "pro time" (pro time is always two words)
PTT		*p*artial *t*hromboplastin *t*ime, a test to determine how fast the blood clots
rales [Fr.]	(răhlz) (rālz)	abnormal respiratory sounds heard on auscultation, indicating some pathologic condition
sodium		salt; an essential chemical element of the body
thorax	(thō′răks)	chest
wheezes		a whistling sound heard on listening to a patient's respirations

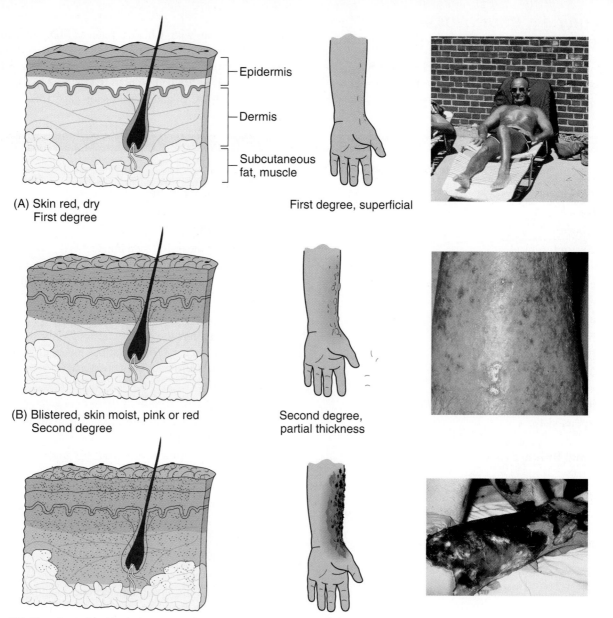

(A) Skin red, dry
First degree

First degree, superficial

(B) Blistered, skin moist, pink or red
Second degree

Second degree,
partial thickness

(C) Charring, skin black, brown, red
Third degree

Third degree, full thickness

Figure QC23-1   Burns Are Usually Referred to as (A) First, (B) Second, or (C) Third Degree (Photos courtesy of The Phoenix Society for Burn Survivors, Inc.)

REPORT 24: HEMATOLOGY CONSULT

Sabar Samaan, an Egyptian gentleman, is referred for hematology consult because of the finding of anemia during a recent hospitalization. A complete exam was done, including lab studies. Copies of the consult were sent to the patient's referring physician and to his primary care physician. See Figure QC24-1, Red Blood Cells, on page 160.

GLOSSARY		
Word	**Phonetic Prounciation**	**Definition**
% sat.		abbreviation for percent *sat*uration of oxygen bound to hemoglobin as measured with a pulse oximeter
adult-onset diabetes mellitus	(dī″ăh-bē′tēz mĕ-lī′tŭs)	also referred to as type 2 diabetes, a condition of excessive amounts of sugar in the blood (hyperglycemia)
CEA		abbreviation for *c*arcino*e*mbryonic *a*ntigen (laboratory test)
endoscopically	(ĕn″dō-skŏp′ĭk-lē)	viewing (examining) inside a body orifice or an internal organ via endoscope
ferritin	(fer′ĭ-tĭn)	an essential iron-apoferritin complex; one method in which iron is stored within the body
Glucophage	(glū′kō-fawzh)	a preparation of metformin, used in type 2 diabetes (trade name)
hemoglobin electrophoresis	(hē-mō-glō′bĭn ē-lĕk-trō-fōr′ē-sĭs)	laboratory test done on red blood cells
hemoglobinopathy	(hē′mō-glō-bĭ-nŏp′ă-thē)	disease condition of the blood (hemoglobin) often resulting in anemia
hepatitis	(hĕp-ă-tī′tĭs)	inflammation of the liver
hypochromic	(hī-pō-krō′mĭk)	disease condition of erythrocytes (red blood cells)
microcytic anemia	(mī″krō-sĭt′-ĭk ă-nē′mē-ah)	any anemia characterized by erythrocytes smaller than normal
Monospot	(mŏn′ō-spŏt)	trade name for a test performed on serum when looking for infectious mononucleosis
plts		abbreviation for platelets (thrombocytes)
Prozac	(prō′zăk)	an antidepressant medication (trade name)
PSA		abbreviation for *p*rostate-*s*pecific *a*ntigen; laboratory test to determine if PSA is present in the prostate gland
retic count	(rē-tĭk′)	abbreviation for *retic*ulocyte count (laboratory test)
serum iron	(sēr′ŭm)	iron found in the serum
target cells		abnormally thin red blood cells seen in certain conditions of anemia
TIBC		abbreviation for *t*otal *i*ron-*b*inding *c*apacity (laboratory test)

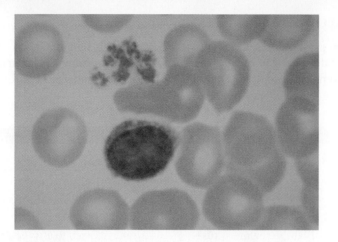

**Figure QC24-1   Photomicrograph of Red Blood Cells with a
White Blood Cell and a Clump of Platelets**

REPORT 25: CORRESPONDENCE

Dr. David Cohen, hematologist, sends a letter to Mr. Sabar Samaan's referring physician (Dr. Austin Whitney) in which Dr. Cohen describes his evaluation, findings, and plan for the patient. A copy of the letter is sent to the patient's primary care physician, Dr. Patrick Keathley. See Figure QC25-1, Spleen.

GLOSSARY		
Word	**Phonetic Prounciation**	**Definition**
occult blood	(ŏ-kŭlt′)	obscure (hidden) blood
thalassemia minor	(thăl-ă-sē′mē-ah)	blood disease sometimes marked by moderate anemia and an enlarged spleen; this form of the disease is often asymptomatic

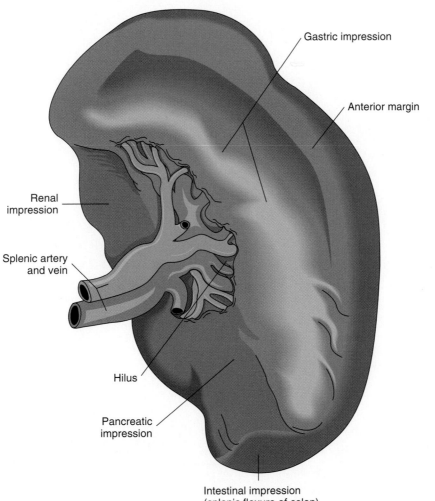

Figure QC25-1   External View of the Spleen

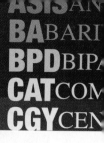
SECTION 6
Skill-Building Exercises

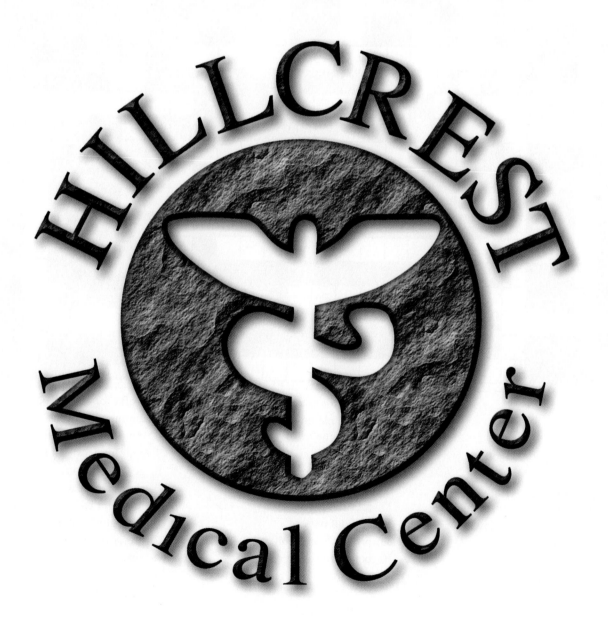

Crossword Puzzle 1

Student _____

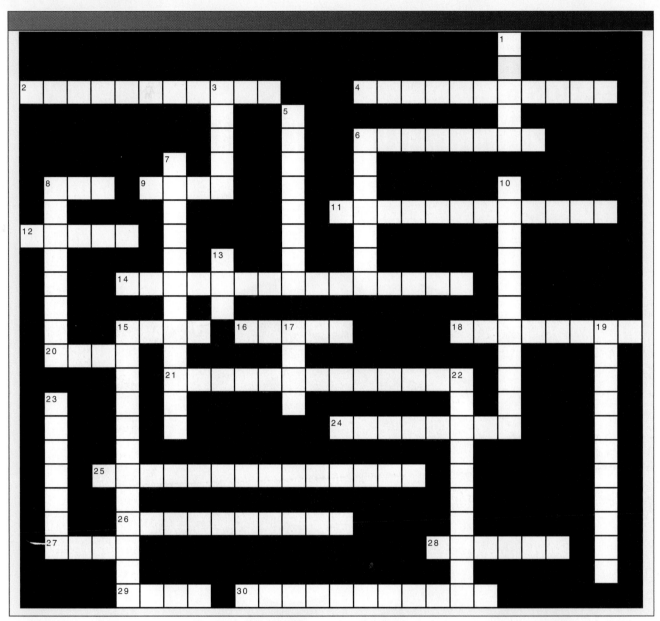

Across

2. affecting both sides
4. pertaining to two joints
6. removal
8. prefix for above, upon
9. prefix for deficient, below
11. inflammation of many nerves
12. not breathing
14. total hysterectomy
15. prefix for near, beside
16. prefix for above, excessive
18. complete separation
20. prefix for before
21. inflammation of one half of the tongue
24. double vision
25. near the esophagus
26. within the skull
27. prefix for within
28. without oxygen
29. prefix for one half, partly
30. before the onset of fever

Down

1. prefix for small
3. prefix for behind, backward
5. uniting together
6. out of normal position
7. painful menstrual flow
8. good digestion
10. slow heartbeat
13. prefix for bad, painful, difficult
15. through the skin
17. prefix for many
19. between the ribs
22. situated above a kidney
23. a newborn infant

Crossword Puzzle 2

Student _____

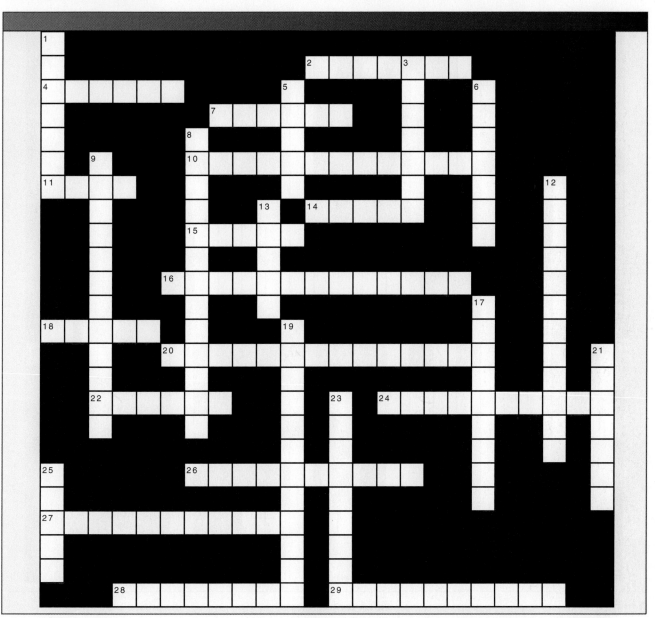

Across

2. abnormal dryness
4. combining form for joint
7. combining form for side
10. suture of the intestine
11. pertaining to the mouth
14. combining form for stone, calculus
15. pertaining to the kidney
16. surgical repair of an artery
18. combining form for tooth
20. constriction of the stomach
22. absence of oxygen
24. destruction of tissue
26. any disease of the bursa
27. any disease of the skull
28. a discharge from the ear
29. incision of a joint

Down

1. combining form for arm
3. combining form for mouth
5. combining form for nerve
6. combining form for pulse
8. hemorrhage from a kidney
9. pertaining to the lips and tongue
12. formation of bone marrow
13. combining form for sacrum
17. an x-ray of the urinary bladder
19. pain in the coccyx
21. combining form for internal organs
23. blood in the urine
25. combining form for cheek

Crossword Puzzle 3

Student _____

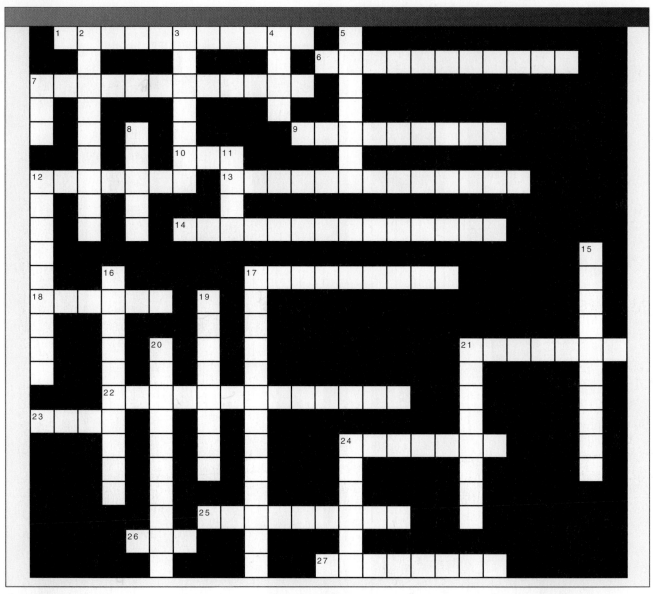

Across

1. pain in the stomach
6. excessive vomiting
7. softening of bone
9. discharge of the menses
10. suffix for specialist
12. absence of the sense of smell
13. study of the eye
14. drooping of the eyelid
17. surgical creation of a new opening in the colon
18. suffix for new opening
21. suffix for treatment
22. suture of a hernia
23. suffix for vision
24. pertaining to the heart
25. bad digestion
26. suffix for little, small
27. lack of strength

Down

2. a minute arterial branch
3. pain in the ear
4. suffix for inflammation
5. difficult breathing
7. suffix for tumor
8. suffix for smell
11. suffix for an instrument used to cut bone
12. dimming of vision
15. spitting blood
16. excessive eating
17. the formation of cartilage
19. inflammation of a bone
20. enlargement of extremities
21. pertaining to the chest
24. suffix for irrigation, washing

Crossword Puzzle 4

Student _____

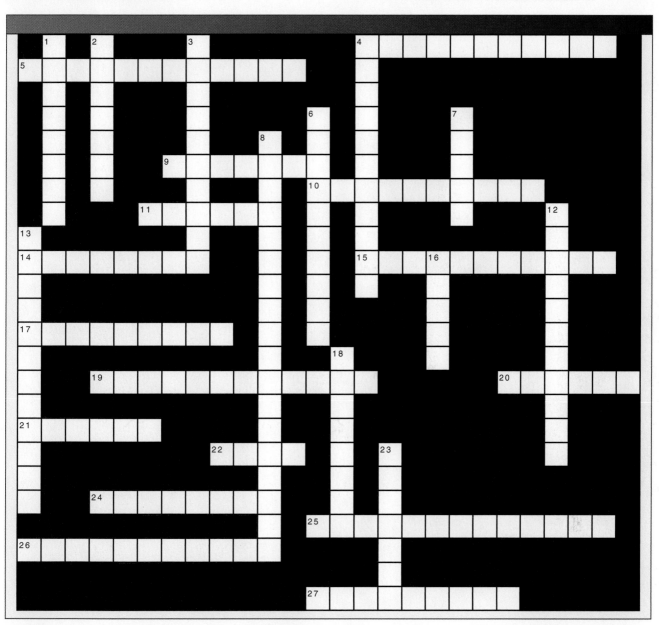

Across

4. abnormally decreased motor function
5. enlargement of one or more of the viscera
9. to cut apart or separate
10. the arrest of bleeding by surgical means
11. the passage of black stools
14. a rattling sound in the lower respiratory tract heard on auscultation
15. situated between the ribs
17. blood in the urine
19. beneath the skin
20. the base of anything
21. chest
22. to bend
24. obstruction of blood to a body part due to a pathological condition
25. surgical removal of a uterine tube
26. surgical removal of an embolus from a blood vessel
27. occurring on both sides

Down

1. closer to any point of reference
2. a vague feeling of bodily discomfort
3. lower chambers of the heart
4. the vomiting of blood
6. pain in a joint
7. pertaining to an opening where the vessels and nerves enter an organ
8. enlargement of the liver and spleen
12. within a vein
13. surgical opening into the trachea
16. accumulation of fluid in intercellular tissue spaces resulting in swelling
18. the presence of fungi in the bloodstream
23. labored breathing

Crossword Puzzle 5

Student _____

Across

1. a rounded and somewhat elevated surface
2. an abnormal respiratory sound
3. enlargement of the spleen
6. the study of the skin
7. the gums
10. painful urination
12. low blood pressure
14. two main arteries that supply blood to the head and neck
18. inflammation of the joints
19. inflammation of the intestine
20. destruction of the surface of the epidermis, which heals without scar tissue
21. difficulty in swallowing
22. a wasting away
23. pertaining to the lumbar region of the spine and the sacrum

Down

1. surgical removal of the gallbladder
4. lying face downward
5. pertaining to the kidney
8. located between two adjoining vertebrae
9. joint disease
10. widely distributed
11. to eliminate as waste matter
12. abnormally increased coloration
13. to surgically remove part of an organ
15. the supporting tissue of an organ
16. redness of the skin
17. a sound heard on auscultation

Proofreading Exercise 6

Student _____ (15 errors)

RADIOLOGY REPORT

Patient Name: Wayne Masten

Hospital No.: 709911

X-ray No.: 03-81938

Admitting Physician: Hannah Sommers, MD

Procedure: PA and lateral chest.

Date: 12/21/- - - -

CLINICAL INFORMATION: Weakness, lethargy. Rule out AIDS, *Pneumocystis* pneumonia. Patient has difficulty breathin and has been unable to gain wait. No IV drug abuse but she admits to promisecuity. Old films are unavailable for comparison.

Findings of underling COPD are noted. The heart size appears normal. The pulmonary vessels, where they can be evaluated, appear unremarkable. Their is no evidence of plural effusion.

Extensive interstitial infiltrates are presnet throughout both lungs. The findings are most consistant with diffused bilateral interstitial pneumonia. I presume we are dealing predominantly with interstitial fibrosis. The lung sare hyperinflated, and there are emphysematous changes in both upper lobe, more prominent on the right.

IMPRESSION
1. COPD with bullous emphysema.
2. Sever diffuse interstitial lung disease, most likely interstitial fibrosis.
3. *Pneumocystis carinii* pneumonia should be considered in the differential diagnosis.

_____
Anne J. Tulsa, MD

ATJ:xx
D:12/21/- - - -
T:12/21/- - - -

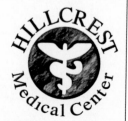

Proofreading Exercise 7

Student _____ (18 errors)

REQUEST FOR CONSULTATION

Patient Name: Victor Peterson

Hospital No.: 973577

Consultant: Mary Wells, MD, Gastroenterology Services

Requesting Physician: Erik Lunderman, MD, Pulmonary/Respiratory Services

Date: 10/16/- - - -

Reason for Consultation: Please evaluate RUQ abdominal pain.

HISTORY: This patient, a 58-year-old male, been seen at the request of his pulmonary/respiratory physician on Friday, October 16, has been admitted to the hospital for elective thorocotomy and decortication for suspected mesothelioma. The patient has a long history of asbestos expo sure, having difficulty with shoulder and arm pain, with the diagnosis of mesothelioma. Two days ago he developed right upper quadrant abdominal pain. The patient has never experienced this type of dyscomfort; he has had no history of acid peptic disease, no known cholelithiasis. He denies fever, chills, hemituria, disurea, or frequency.

PHYSICAL EXAMINATION being done at this time is limited to the abdomin where bowel sounds are present and normal. There are no discreet mass felt. There is fullness in the right upper quadrant, and the patient does exhibit some minimal tenderness to palpation in the right upper quadrant. The patient has being a febrile. Ultrasound of the gall bladder does show cholelithiasis with a borderling common duct.

DISCUSSION: At the present time the patient is known to have stones. I suspect his discomfort is from either an episodes of cholecystitis nor choledocholithiasis. I would suspect that livor function studies may be helpful in suggesting the presents of choledocholithiasis. We will make arrangements for the LFTs and possible sphincterotomy.

IMPRESSION
1. Status post resection of mesothelioma.
2. Cholelithiasis, rule out choledocholithiasis.

(Continued)

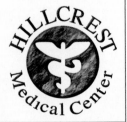

DISCHARGE SUMMARY
Patient Name: Victor Peterson
Hospital No.: 973577
Date of Consult: 10/16/ - - - -
Page 2

Thank you very much for allowing us to participate in the care of your patient. We will follow her along with you as necessary.

_____

Mary Wells, MD

MW:xx
D:10/16/- - - -
T:10/17/- - - -

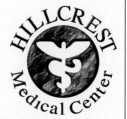

Proofreading Exercise 8

Student _____ (21 errors)

HISTORY AND PHYSICAL EXAMINATION

Patient Name: Maria Elena Ramirez

Hospital No.: 158376

Room No.: 532

Date of Admission: 10/20/- - - -

Admitting Physician: Hal Seggerman, MD

Admitting Diagnosis: Rule out adenomyosis of uterus.

CHIEF COMPLAIN: Exceedingly heavy and painfully menses.

PRESENT ILLNESS: Patient is a 35-year-old, mildly obese Hispanic female, gravida 5, para 4-1-0-4, whose younger child is 13 years old. Patient states that over the past one years or so she has had increasing difficulty with moodiness, depression, generalized fatigue, weight gain, and bloating premenstrually. The symptoms described preceed her menses by about a weak. She was seen by another physician and diagnosed as having menstrual endometrium.

PAST SURGICAL HISTORY: She has had DNCs on two occasions five or six years ago for what sounds like menorrhagia/metrorrhagia. A sterilization procedure was done afterbirth of her last child.

ALLERGIES, PAST HISTORY, AND MEDICATIONS: The patient is allergic to Ergotrate an Iodine, especially in the forum of IVP die. Her only medication at present is Motrin used p.r.n. menstrual cramps. She has had the usual childhood diseases with no sequelae, no serious adult illnesses, no similar problems in her remote passed.

PHYSICAL EXAMINATION: VITAL SIGN: Completely within normal limits. HEENT: Normocephalic. PERRLA. NECK: No crepitus. Trachea is midline. No JVD. BREASTS are pendulous with a monilial appearing rash between the breasts. No masses, tenderness, or discharge. Areola are darkly pigmented. ABDOMEN: Fatty abdominal apron with a well-heeled scar at the sight of her sterilization procedure. No hepatosplenomegaly. Positive bowel sounds. PELVIC/RECTAL: Introduction of speculum reveals the cervix to be multiparous and clean. No vaginal wall lesions are noted. On by manual exam, uterus is exquisitely tender to

(Continued)

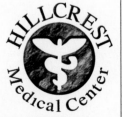

HISTORY AND PHYSICAL EXAMINATION
Patient Name: Maria Elena Ramirez
Hospital No.: 15837
Date of Admission: 10/20/ - - - -
Page 2

compression and is retroversion in position. Adnexa are negative for masses but are moderately tender. BUS negative. Rectal exam confirmatory with some internal and external hemorrhoid. SKIN: Patient has had some itching between her breasts and on her inner thighs due to apparent Monilia. NEUROLOGIC: No focale deficits.

IMPRESSING
1. Cyclic edema inadequately compensated.
2. Probable adenomyosis of the uterus.
3. Monilia.
4. Internal and external hemorrhoids.

_____

Hal Seggerman, MD

HS:xx
D:10/20/- - - -
T:10/21/- - - -

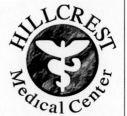

Proofreading Exercise 9

Student _____ (19 errors)

HISTORY AND PHYSICAL EXAMINATION

Patient Name: Christina Youngblood

Hospital No.: 712102

Room No.: 418

Date of Admission: 06/24/- - - -

Admitting Physician: Cynthia Richards, MD

Admitting Diagnosis: Cystocele, prolapsed uterus, B9 cyst of vulva.

CHIEF COMPLAINT: Painful menstrual flew; urinary incontinence.

PRESENT ILLNESS: This 38-year-old Native American female presented with increased menstrual flow and stress urinary incontinence over the last too years. No other complaints.

PAST MEDICAL HISTORY: Essentially negative except for pyelonefritis as a child with no sequelae. Scarlet fever at age 19 with subsequent tonsilectomy. Has had "sinus trouble" in the past, which cleared after she stopped smoking. (Smoked approximate a pack a day between the ages of 16 and 26 years.)

MEDICATIONS: None. No allergies save for a reaction to ASA.

FAMILY HISTORY: Mother has COPD. Father has hearing lost and elevated cholesterol. One sibling with hearing loss. Maternal aunt with diabetes mellitos, adult onset.

SOCIAL HISTORY: Divorced. Formal smoker (see PMH). Drinks wine socially. Two daughter, aged 6 and 15, in good healthy.

PHYSICAL EXAMINATION: In general, a Well-developed, well-nourished, obese American Indian woman with stable vitals. HEENT: Normocephalic, atraumatic. No neck masses. CHEST: Clear to PNA. HEART: Not enlarge, regular rate and rhythm. No murmurs. BREASTS: No masses. ABDOMEN: Soft, nontender. No organomegaly, PELVIC: Six-centimeter superficial cyst, right upper labia minora. Cystocele.

(Continued)

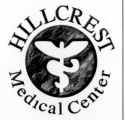

HISTORY AND PHYSICAL EXAMINATION
Patient Name: Christina Youngblood
Hospital No.: 712102
Date of Admission: 06/26/ - - - -
Page 2

Uterus normal sized with mile prolapse. Cervix oval, clean. Adnexa, cul de sac clean.
RECTAL: Confirmatory. EXTREMITIES: Pulses 2+, no edema. NEUROLOGIC
EXAM: Cranial nerves II thru XII intact as tested.

DISPOSITION: Admit for possible urinary bladder repair and hysterectomy.

_____
Cynthia Richards, MD

CR:xx
D:06/24/- - - -
T:06/25/- - - -

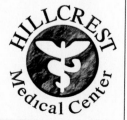

Proofreading Exercise 10

Student _____ (16 errors)

DISCHARGE SUMMARY

Patient Name: Kurt G. Kinsey

Hospital No.: 314988

Admitted: 07/21/- - - -

Discharged: 07/26/- - - -

Consultations: None.

Procedures: Bilateral correcton of hallux valgus with osteotomy, right; Akin procedure, left.

Complications: None.

Admitting Diagnoses: Bilateral hallux valgus.

This 15-year-old young men was admitted for scheduled surgery as listed above.

DIAGNOSTIC DATA ON ADMISSION: WBC 6.5, RBC 4.53, hemoglobin 14.1, hematocrit 41, MCV 92, MCH 31.1, MCHC 3.2, platelets 26100; differential, 42 polys, 40 limps, 3 bands, 10 monos, 5 eos. Urinalysis, clear yellow with specific gravity 1.025, PH 5, glucose negative, keytones negative, bilirubin negative. No red cells, no white cells, urobilinogen normal. RPR nonreactive. Postoperative chest film normally.

HOSPITAL COURSE: Patient response to anesthesia uneventfully. Postoperatively patient was hemodynamically stable, afebrile. Physical therapy was instituted during hospital stayed. Therapist taught the patient to use crutches, including on stares and at curbs. Patient did well postoperatively and with the visual therapy.

DISCHARGE DIAGNOSIS: Bilateral hallux valgus, corrected.

(Continued)

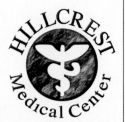

DISCHARGE SUMMARY
Patient Name: Kurt G. Kinsey
Hospital No.: 31498
Discharge Date: 07/26/ - - - -
Page 2

DISCHARGE INSTRUCTIONS: He was discharged on postoperative day five in
improved condition to be seen in the office or dressing check in one week. He was
given Tylenol No. 3 p.r.n. pain. Diet regular. Activities: Crutches, no weightbearing,
keep lower limbs iced and elevation as much as possible. Patient voiced
understanding of the plan as described above. Both he and his parents agreed to the
plan and scheduled followup.

_____

Bill Perry, MD

BB:xx
D:07/26/- - - -
T:08/02/- - - -

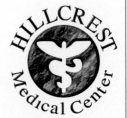

Appendix

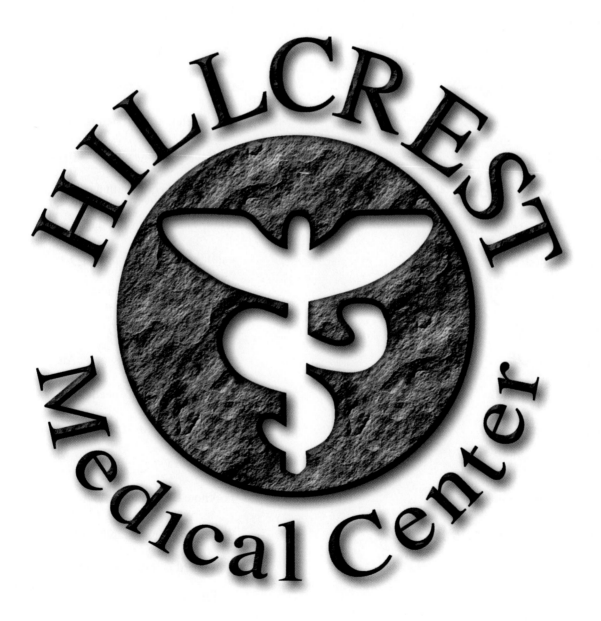

Proofreader's Marks

DEFINED		EXAMPLES

DEFINED

Paragraph ¶

Insert a character ∧

Delete ℓ

Do not change *stet* or ....

Transpose tr

Move to the left [

Move to the right]

No paragraph no ¶

Delete and close up ℓ̂

Set in caps *caps* or ≡

Set in lower case *lc*

Insert a period ⊙

Quotation marks ⸌⸍ ⸌⸍

Comma ⸜

Insert space #

Apostrophe ⸜

Hyphen =

Close up ◡

Use superior figure ⌄

Set in italic *ital.* or ___

Move up ⌐¬

Move down ⌊⌋

EXAMPLES

¶ Begin a new paragraph at this point. Insᵉrt a letter here.

Delete these words. Disregard the previous correction. To transpose is to around turn.

[Move this copy to the left.

] Move this copy to the right.

no ¶ Do not begin a new paragraph here. Delete the hyphen from pre-ê mpt and close up the space.

≡ a sentence begins with a capital letter. This Word should not be capitalized. Insert a period⊙

" Quotation marks and a comma should be placed here he said.

Space between these words. An apostrophe is whats needed here.

Add a hyphen to African American. Close up the extra spa ce.

Footnote this sentence. Set the words, sine qua non, in italics.

This word is too low. That word is too high.

Challenging Medical Words, Phrases, Prefixes

Each of the following words and abbreviations can be difficult or confusing. Some sound alike yet have different meanings, whereas others do not sound alike but are often used and spelled incorrectly. When listening to dictation, MTs should be aware of regional accent pronunciation as well as foreign accent pronunciation. Be prepared to spell, transcribe, and use *each* of the following terms and abbreviations correctly.

affect—noun; a state of mind or mood; countenance

affect—verb; to influence, to produce an effect on

effect—noun; result, impression

effect—verb; to result in, bring about, to accomplish

ala nasi—singular noun meaning naris or opening of the nasal cavity

alae nasi—plural noun meaning nares or openings of the nasal cavity

ante—prefix meaning before, in front of, prior, earlier

anti—prefix meaning against, opposite, over

anterior—in front of, forward part of, toward the head

inferior—below, beneath, directed downward, lower surface

interior—inside, inward, inner part or cavity

appose—to place side by side or next to; before, beside, or on

oppose—to place opposite or against something, so as to provide resistance, counterbalance, or contrast

arteritis—inflammation of an artery.

arthritis—inflammation of a joint

aura—subjective evidence of the beginning of either a seizurelike episode or a migraine headache

aural—relating to the ears or to an aura

oral—relating to the mouth

auxiliary—subordinate, secondary

axillary—referring to the underarm area (sometimes temperature is taken here)

bases—plural of basis

basis—the lower, basic, or fundamental part of an object

bile—fluid secreted by the liver

bowel—intestine

Betagan—an ophthalmologic medication

Betagen—a surgical scrub, antiseptic ointment, or a vitamin supplement

bisect—to cut in half

resect—to cut out a large portion

transect—to cut across

dissect—to cut up, as at autopsy (note the double "s")

caliber—the diameter of a hollow, tubular structure (like a bullet)

caliper—instrument used for measuring diameters, like pelvic diameters

cancer—cellular tumor, usually malignant

carcinoma—malignant new growth (used in the same way as cancer)

CA—abbreviation for carcinoma or cancer but can also stand for cardiac arrest, coronary artery, and other phrases

Ca—chemical symbol for calcium only

callous—adjective meaning hard or bony

callus—noun meaning bone

Carrisyn (generic is acemannan)—an antiviral AIDS drug

Carrasyn Hydrogel (brand name)—a wound dressing, over the counter

chord—a musical word

cord—an anatomic word, e.g., spinal cord

cor—an anatomic word, the heart

cirrhosal—adjective describing a diseased liver

serosal—adjective describing a membrane covering certain cavities of the body

clavicle—collarbone

pedicle—stalk

coarse—rough

course—route, plan

defer—to put off or delay, as in "exam was deferred"

differ—to be unalike or distinct; different

diffuse—adjective meaning scattered, not localized, e.g., diffuse infiltrates

defuse—verb meaning to make a situation less harmful, to calm a crisis diploic—adjective meaning double

diploë—noun meaning loose bony tissue between the cranial bones

discreet—showing good judgment, prudent (not necessarily a medical word)

discrete—made up of separate parts, not blended; e.g., a discrete mass (NOTE: Discrete and separate both end in "te.")

disease—morbid process with train of symptoms

sign—evidence of disease that is seen (objective)

symptom—evidence of disease not seen (subjective)

syndrome—a set of symptoms

diverticulum, datum, and medium are each singular nouns taking singular verbs

diverticula, data, and media are each plural nouns—don't forget the plural verb

DNC—did not come

D&C—dilation and curettage

efflux—outward flow

reflux—backward or return flow

endogenous—growing, developing, or originating from within

exogenous—developing or originating from the outside, e.g., exogenous obesity

enterocleisis—closure of an intestinal wound

enteroclysis—injection of a nutrient or medicinal liquid into the bowel

Eurax—a dermatologic cream, ointment

Urex—a urologic tablet, anti-infective

excise—to cut out or off

incise—to cut into

extirpation—to remove entirely, as in extirpation of varicose veins

extubation—to remove a tube, like a nasogastric tube, from a patient

expiration—synonym for death

fecal sac versus thecal sac—theca is an enclosing case or sheath, and both are good phrases

fundus—bottom or base; the part of a hollow organ farthest from its mouth, e.g., the fundus of the stomach

fungus—any one of a class of mushrooms, yeasts, molds

en bloc—in a lump, whole

in situ—in its normal place, confined to the site of origin

in toto—totally

in vivo—within the living body

in vitro—within a test tube (glass)

glans—(singular) a small, rounded mass of glandlike body, e.g., end of penis

glands—(plural) aggregation of cells specialized to secrete or excrete

graft—tissue for implantation (grafting)

graph—a written record, diagram

grasp—grab hold of or seize, as with a surgical instrument

gravida—a pregnant woman (gravida 1 = primigravida)

multiparous—having had two or more pregnancies resulting in viable offspring (para 2 or para 3, etc.)

nulligravida—never having been pregnant

nulliparous—never having given birth to a viable infant

(NOTE: Gravida 5, para 3-1-1-3 refers to a woman who has been pregnant five times, resulting in three full-term deliveries, one premature birth, one abortion or miscarriage, and three living children.

HNP—herniated nucleus pulposus

H&P—history and physical

hypo—prefix meaning beneath, under, or deficient

hyper—prefix meaning above, beyond, or excessive

illicit—adjective meaning illegal, as in illicit drugs

elicit—verb meaning to bring out, as to elicit a response or reaction

inflamed, inflammatory, inflammation—same root word; note the spelling difference

ilium—bone (iliac crest)

ileum—portion of the small intestine

ileus—disease (obstruction of small intestine)

(NOTE: There is both an iliac artery and an iliac vein.)

inter—prefix meaning situated or occurring between

intra—prefix meaning situated or occurring within

infra—prefix meaning situated or occurring beneath

intubated—having had a tube inserted (as into the larynx for providing oxygen)

incubated—placed in an optimal situation for development

lavage—to wash out or irrigate

gavage—forced feeding, especially through a tube

lineal—pertaining to the spleen, as in gastrolineal ligament

renal—pertaining to the kidneys

ligament—a band of tissue connecting bones, supporting viscera

ligature—a thread or wire (suture) for tying vessels

ligate—a verb meaning to sew, tie, or bind with ligature, as after a surgical procedure

liver—the largest gland in the body

livor—the discoloration of the skin on the dependent parts of a corpse

livid—discolored as from a contusion, congestion, or cyanosis

loose—adjective meaning not tight, as in loose clothes

lose—verb meaning to miss from a customary place, as in "Did you lose the book?"

malleus (pl. mallei)—pertaining to the outermost and largest of the three bones in the ear

malleolus (pl. malleoli)—pertaining to the bony prominences on either side of the ankle joint

melena—blood in the stool, remember *melenic stools* is a proper phrase

melanin—dark brown to black pigment

melanotic—pertaining to the presence of melanin or dark pigment in the skin, hair, etc., and has nothing to do with stool

metacarpal—relating to the hand

metatarsal—relating to the foot between the instep and the toes

mucus—noun meaning the free slime of the mucous membrane

mucous—adjective meaning pertaining to or resembling mucus

occur/recur and occurrence/recurrence—something either occurs or recurs; we have an occurrence or a recurrence. (Remember, "reocur" and "reoccurrence" are *not* acceptable, even if dictated. Transcribe recur or recurrence instead.)

ophthalmologist—a physician specializing in the care of the eyes; note spelling, as "ophthal" is often mispronounced and misspelled

os (pl. ora)—the mouth; any opening into a hollow organ or canal; example, cervical os or medication taken per os

os (pl. ossa)—bone; example, os pubis (pubic bone) or ossa cranii (cranial bones)

ostium—(pl. ostia) a small opening

ostiomeatal—*not* osteo, it denotes an opening and has nothing to do with bone

palpation—to touch or feel, examine with the hand(s)

palpitation—rapid and/or irregular pulsations of the heart

para—prefix meaning beside, beyond

peri—prefix meaning around

perineum—genital area, perineal area (between anus and scrotum or vulva)

peritoneum—covering of viscera, lining of abdominopelvic wall

peroneal—pertaining to the fibula, lateral side of the leg, or to the tissues present there

plane—a flat surface

plain—unadorned

pleural—referring to the pleural cavity

plural—meaning more than one

prostate—the male gland surrounding the urethra

prostrate—overcome (prostrate with grief) or lying in a horizontal position

proximal—nearest, closer to any point of reference, a location

approximate—verb meaning to bring close together, as to approximate the edges of a wound

approximately—adverb meaning estimation

pruritus—noun meaning an itchy skin condition

purulent—adjective meaning containing, consisting of, or forming pus, as in a purulent wound

radicle—an anatomic word, the radicles are the smallest branches

radical—going to the root or source of disease, as in radical dissection at surgery

regimen—strictly regulated scheme of diet, exercise, medication, therapy, or training

regime—same as above but pronounced and spelled differently; also used to refer to a government

regiment—a military unit; to organize rigidly

retroperitoneal—adverb meaning behind the peritoneum (a direction)

reperitonealize—verb meaning to cover again with peritoneum

shoddy—inferior goods, hastily or poorly done

shotty—like shot, lead pellets used in shotguns (usually used in reference to lymph nodes, e.g., shotty nodes)

sulfa—pertaining to the sulfonamides, the sulfa drugs

sulfur—brimstone, an element, the symbol for which is S

tendon—noun meaning a band of connective tissue

tendinous—adjective meaning resembling a tendon

tendinitis—noun meaning inflammation of a tendon or tendons (note spelling)

tenia (pl. teniae)—any anatomic bandlike structure

tinea—ringworm, which is a fungus

tinnitus—abnormal noises in the ears, such as ringing or booming or whistling

tonsil, tonsillectomy—same root word; note spelling difference

umbo (pl. umbones)—a round projection, an orthopedic term

umbonate—knoblike

ureter—tube from kidney to bladder; there is a left and a right ureter

urethra—tube carrying urine out of the body; one per person

vagus—noun meaning the tenth cranial nerve or vagus nerve

valgus—adjective meaning bent outward, twisted, deformed

vesicle—little blister or sac

vesical—urinary bladder *only*

villus (pl. villi)—noun meaning little protrusion

villous—adjective meaning shaggy with soft hairs

(NOTE: There could be a villous villus.)

womb—the uterus

wound—trauma to the body

xerosis—dryness

cirrhosis—liver disease

Proper terms for people of different ages include

neonates or newborns = birth to 1 month of age

infants = 1 month to 2 years of age

children = 2 years to 13 years of age (also boys and girls)

adolescents = 13 years through 17 years of age

adults = 18 years and older (also men and women)

Inflammation is diagnosed when all of the following elements, often referred to as the cardinal signs of inflammation, are present.

calor (heat)

dolor (pain)

rubor (redness)

tumor (swelling)

Reference material used in developing this list includes Dorland's Illustrated Medical Dictionary, *30th edition;* Stedman's Medical Dictionary, *26th edition;* AMA Manual of Style, *9th edition;* Gregg Reference Manual, *9th edition; and* The AAMT Book of Style, *2nd edition.*

Sample Patient History Form

Patient Name:_____   Date:_____

	DOCTOR OR THERAPIST USE ONLY

1. PLEASE CHECK THE AREA OF YOUR MAJOR COMPLAINT.
   ☐ HEADACHE   ☐ NECK   ☐ BETWEEN SHOULDERS   ☐ LOW BACK
   ☐ SHOULDER   ☐ HIP   ☐ ARM   ☐ LEG

2. HOW DID THIS EPISODE BEGIN (CHECK APPROPRIATE ANSWER)?
   ☐ LIFTING   ☐ HIT IN BACK
   ☐ TWISTING   ☐ AUTO ACCIDENT → DATE OF INJURY:_____
   ☐ PUSHING   ☐ ON THE JOB → DATE OF INJURY:_____
   ☐ PULLING   ☐ UNKNOWN
   ☐ BENDING   ☐ OTHER:_____
   _____

3. WHEN DID THIS EPISODE OF PAIN BEGIN?_____

4. HAVE YOU HAD A SIMILAR EPISODE BEFORE?   ☐ YES   ☐ NO

5. WHAT TESTS HAVE YOU HAD AND WHAT ARE THE RESULTS?
   1.
   2.
   3.
   4.

6. LIST DOCTORS AND THERAPISTS YOU HAVE SEEN, AND THE RESULTS.
   1.
   2.
   3.
   4.

7. WHAT HAVE YOU BEEN TOLD IS WRONG?
   ☐ PINCHED NERVE   ☐ ARTHRITIS
   ☐ SLIPPED DISC   ☐ NOT TOLD
   ☐ PULLED MUSCLE
   ☐ OTHER:_____

8. FOR YOUR NECK OR BACK, HAVE YOU EVER HAD
   ☐ HOSPITALIZATION   ☐ BONE SCAN
   ☐ X-RAYS   ☐ MYELOGRAM
   ☐ CAT SCAN   ☐ EMG
   ☐ MRI SCAN   ☐ NONE
   ☐ OTHER:_____

9. HAVE YOU TAKEN ANY MEDICINE FOR THIS PROBLEM?
   ☐ NONE   ☐ FELDENE   ☐ IBUPROFEN
   ☐ MOTRIN   ☐ MECLOMEN   ☐ ALEVE
   ☐ NALFON   ☐ ORUDIS   ☐ ASPRIN
   ☐ NAPROSYN   ☐ ORUVAIL   ☐ TYLENOL
   ☐ CLINORIL   ☐ RELAFEN   ☐ CORTISONE: STEROIDS
   ☐ INDOCIN   ☐ LODINE   PREDNISONE
   ☐ TOLECTIN   ☐ ADVIL   DECADRON
   ☐ OTHER:_____   MEDROL

10.

HAVE YOU HAD	YES	NO	BETTER	WORSE	SAME
PHYSICAL THERAPY	☐	☐	☐	☐	☐
CORSET OR BRACE	☐	☐	☐	☐	☐
CHIROPRACTIC	☐	☐	☐	☐	☐
MASSAGE	☐	☐	☐	☐	☐
BACK SURGERY	☐	☐	☐	☐	☐
ACUPUNCTURE	☐	☐	☐	☐	☐
CORTISONE SHOT	☐	☐	☐	☐	☐

Patient Name:_____

11. USE THESE SYMBOLS TO SHOW AREA ON THE DRAWINGS WHERE YOU HAVE SYMPTOMS.

>>>ACHE   ☐ ☐ NUMBNESS   ☐ ☐ PINS AND NEEDLES   X X BURNING   //// STABBING

RIGHT

LEFT   RIGHT

LEFT

R   L

RIGHT   LEFT   LEFT

RIGHT

R   L

---

12. ARE YOUR SYMPTOMS GETTING   ☐ BETTER   ☐ SAME   ☐ WORSE

13. PLEASE CHECK ONE ANSWER IF IT APPLIES TO YOU.
     ☐ BACK (NECK) PAIN IS WORSE THAN LEG (ARM) PAIN
     ☐ BACK (NECK) PAIN EQUALS LEG (ARM) PAIN
     ☐ LEG (ARM) PAIN IS WORSE THAN BACK (NECK) PAIN

14. PLEASE CHECK <u>ALL</u> OF THE FOLLOWING THAT BEST DESCRIBE YOUR PAIN.
     ☐ CONSTANT   ☐ WAKES YOU UP AT NIGHT
     ☐ DAILY   ☐ WORSE WITH COUGH OR SNEEZE
     ☐ WORSE IN MORNING   ☐ WORSE WITH ACTIVITY

15. CHECK THE APPROPRIATE BOXES REGARDING YOUR PAIN.

	WORSE	BETTER	NO CHANGE
SITTING	☐	☐	☐
STANDING	☐	☐	☐
GETTING UP FROM SITTING	☐	☐	☐
BENDING FORWARD	☐	☐	☐
LEANING BACKWARD	☐	☐	☐
LIFTING	☐	☐	☐
WALKING	☐	☐	☐
REST	☐	☐	☐
LYING ON BACK	☐	☐	☐
LYING ON STOMACH	☐	☐	☐
MENSTRUAL PERIODS	☐	☐	☐

16. HAVE YOU LOST CONTROL OF YOUR BOWELS OR BLADDER?
     ☐ YES   ☐ NO

DOCTOR OR THERAPIST USE ONLY

The Lund Browder Chart

The Burn Extent Estimator is a convenient method of estimating the percentage of a patient's burn, the total surface area of the patient's body in square feet, and the approximate surface area of the burn, in square feet.

Shade the burn areas on the figures below, and use the table to estimate the percentage of the burn.

Area	Age—Years					% 2°	% 3°	% Total
	0–1	1–4	5–9	10–15	Adult			
Head	19	17	13	10	7			
Neck	2	2	2	2	2			
Ant. Trunk	13	13	13	13	13			
Post. Trunk	13	13	13	13	13			
R. Buttock	2 ½	2 ½	2 ½	2 ½	2 ½			
L. Buttock	2 ½	2 ½	2 ½	2 ½	2 ½			
Genitalia	1	1	1	1	1			
R.U. Arm	4	4	4	4	4			
L.U. Arm	4	4	4	4	4			
R.L. Arm	3	3	3	3	3			
L.L. Arm	3	3	3	3	3			
R. Hand	2 ½	2 ½	2 ½	2 ½	2 ½			
L. Hand	2 ½	2 ½	2 ½	2 ½	2 ½			
R. Thigh	5 ½	6 ½	8 ½	8 ½	9 ½			
L. Thigh	5 ½	6 ½	8 ½	8 ½	9 ½			
R. Leg	5	5	5 ½	6	7			
L. Leg	5	5	5 ½	6	7			
R. Foot	3 ½	3 ½	3 ½	3 ½	3 ½			
L. Foot	3 ½	3 ½	3 ½	3 ½	3 ½			
					TOTAL			

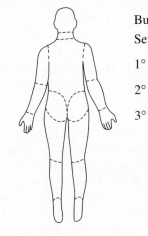

Burn Evaluation
Severity of Burn

1° =

2° =

3° =

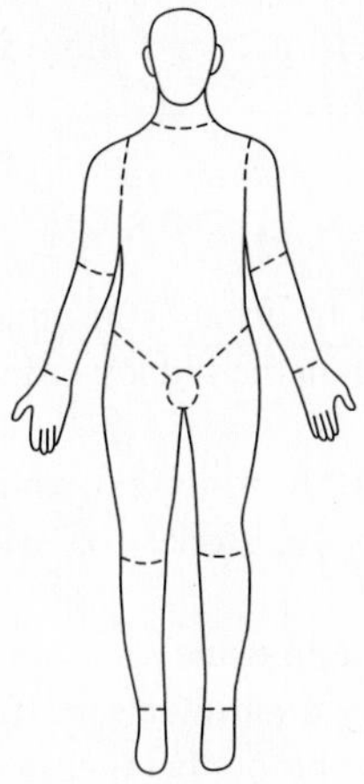

Laboratory Test Information

COMPLETE BLOOD COUNT (CBC)

Segmented neutrophils (segs), basophils, (basos), eosinophils (eos), bands, lymphocytes (lymphs), and monocytes (monos) represent different types of white blood cells. Counting the types of WBCs is known as the white blood cell differential count, often dictated as the "diff." Analyzing the patterns of the differential can give information about many diseases. A "shift to the left" indicates an increase in the percentage of unsegmented (immature) neutrophils, also called band cells or bands. A "shift to the right" indicates an increase in the percentage of multisegmented (mature) neutrophils, also called segs.

hemoglobin (Hgb) **hematocrit (Hct)**	The H&H results give different measures of red blood cell volume. Low levels indicate anemia. Hemoglobin is reported in grams or g/dL; hematocrit is reported in percent.
white blood cells (WBCs)	White cells (leukocytes) fight infection, and high levels can indicate infection. Low levels can be due to medication or even bone marrow suppression.
red blood cells (RBCs)	Red cells are erythrocytes, and this is a measure of red blood cells in a certain volume of blood.
platelets	Platelets are components essential for coagulation (clotting).
MCV, MCH, MCHC	Known as the red blood cell indices, the MCH, MCV, and MCHC describe the size of the red blood cells and the amount of hemoglobin in the red cells. For example, iron deficiency anemia and pernicious anemia would have different indices. The initials stand for mean corpuscular volume (MCV), mean corpuscular hemoglobin (MCH), and mean corpuscular hemoglobin concentration (MCHC).

URINALYSIS (UA)

Testing some chemical reactions in the urine and looking at centrifuged debris (sediment) under the microscope gives information about different diseases, including those of the kidney and urinary bladder.

glucose (sugar)	The presence of glucose may indicate diabetes mellitus.
protein	The presence of protein may indicate kidney disease but is also seen with recent exercise, dehydration, heart failure, and multiple myeloma.
specific gravity	This is a measurement of the concentration of urine, being low after consuming abundant fluids and being high with dehydration.
pH	This measures the acidity of urine, always transcribed pH.

MICROSCOPIC URINALYSIS

White blood cells (WBCs) in urine seen under a microscope can be due to infection in the kidney or in the urinary bladder.

Red blood cells (RBCs) in urine seen under a microscope may be due to infection, stones, or even a malignancy.

The presence of bacteria in urine seen under a microscope may indicate a urinary tract infection. If a specimen has been sitting out for a time before being tested, however, bacteria could be present from just sitting too long with no true urinary tract infection present.

PROTHROMBIN TIME WITH INR AND THE PARTIAL THROMBOPLASTIN TIME

The PT/PTT blood tests are used to track anticoagulation, and the results are often dictated together. The prothrombin time or pro time (PT) can be used to keep track of Coumadin levels. The partial thromboplastin time (PTT) can be used to keep track of heparin levels. Coumadin and heparin are both blood thinners. PT/PTT results can be abnormal with blood abnormalities, liver disease, hemophilia, etc.

The PT and INR results (International Normalized Ratio) may be dictated without the PTT. (Example: PT is 16.5 seconds with an INR of 1.4%.) The INR is a method of improving prothrombin time tests despite variations in the properties of different batches of thromboplastin used in the test.

SEDIMENTATION RATE (SED RATE)

A nonspecific test that indicates inflammation anywhere in the body, the sed rate may be elevated in the presence of infection, malignancy, trauma, and/or certain types of rheumatism. Like an elevated temperature, the sedimentation rate indicates a problem but defines neither the location nor the type of problem. This test is also known as the ESR (erythrocyte sedimentation rate).

THYROID FUNCTION TESTS (TFTs)

T_3, T_4 (sometimes transcribed T3, T4), and TSH are the usual screening tests for thyroid disease.

T_3 (triiodothyronine) is an organic, iodine-containing hormone compound secreted in small amounts by the thyroid gland.

T_4 (thyroxine) is the principal hormone manufactured by the thyroid gland. If elevated, it may indicate an overactive thyroid (hyperthyroidism). If low, underactive thyroid disease (hypothyroidism) may be the cause.

TSH (thyroid-stimulating hormone) is manufactured by the pituitary gland and directs the thyroid gland to either increase or decrease production of thyroxine (T_4). In the usual form of hypothyroidism, the T_4 is low, and the TSH is high. Low T_4 *and* TSH levels may indicate hypothyroidism secondary to pituitary disease. T_3, T_4, and TSH may be decreased by either an acute or a chronic illness, by fasting, or by severe stress.

PROSTATE SPECIFIC ANTIGEN (PSA)

Prostate specific antigen is a substance produced in the prostate gland. Normal levels are between 0 and 4. The most common cause of an elevated PSA (>4) is prostate enlargement, known as benign prostatic hyperplasia (BPH). An elevated PSA, however, can also indicate prostatic cancer. Being a nonspecific test, a diagnosis may require additional studies, including ultrasound and/or needle biopsy of the prostate.

CHEMISTRY PROFILE (CHEM PROFILE)

A chemistry profile is a group of blood studies that provide information about internal bodily function and disease. It is an effective and economical study using a small blood sample and performed on a machine (sometimes called a SMAC or a Coulter) that runs the tests simultaneously. A chemistry profile is known as a "screening procedure" and is designed to uncover common diseases that might be missed on physical examination. It usually provides no definite answers, since most diagnoses require more specific tests and correlation with the physician's history and physical exam. The blood tests and their significance are discussed below.

Blood Test	Significance
glucose	Sugar in the blood, high levels of which can indicate diabetes mellitus.
cholesterol cholesterol/HDL trigylcerides cholesterol/LDL	Known as the lipid (fat) profile, the pattern of results provides information about fat metabolism. Abnormal patterns can indicate a tendency for coronary artery disease. Generally, lower levels of cholesterol, HDL, triglycerides, and LDL are ideal. With HDL, the "good" cholesterol, however, higher levels are better than lower levels.
blood urea nitrogen and creatinine	The BUN and creatinine measure kidney function; their results are usually dictated together.
uric acid	Commonly high with gout, the uric acid level is abnormal in kidney disease, with tissue breakdown, dehydration, and in other disease conditions.
calcium and phosphorus	Abnormal levels can indicate disease of the bone, parathyroid gland, kidneys, and other diseases.

Blood Test	Significance
bilirubin, alkaline phosphatase, AST (SGOT), ALT (SGPT), LDH, and GGPT	This group of chemistry tests is commonly referred to as a liver function panel or the liver function tests (LFTs). The bilirubin is a yellow pigment and can be abnormal with liver and gallbladder disease plus certain blood diseases. The alkaline phosphatase (often dictated alk phos) is an enzyme that indicates bone disease, cancer, or other disease. AST, ALT, and LDL are enzymes that can be abnormal with liver, muscle, or heart disease. (AST and ALT are preferred usage over SGOT and SGPT, but you may hear any one of them on dictation. You should type what you hear.) GGPT distinguishes liver disease from other disease.
protein and albumin-globulin ratio	These provide a picture of general nutrition, liver function, and acute or chronic inflammation.
sodium, potassium, chloride, and bicarbonate (electrolytes)	This group of four chemistry tests is known as the electrolytes (often dictated "lytes"). They can be abnormal with kidney disease, liver or respiratory failure, dehydration, and diuretic therapy (water pills).

Chemistry terminology also heard on dictation includes

BMP (basic metabolic profile)

CMP (complete metabolic profile)

SMAC-8 (8 chemistry tests)

SMAC-21 (21 chemistry tests)

NOTE: Each of the above descriptions is meant to provide some basic information about the many tests done in the clinical laboratory. Normal results do not always assure good health; abnormal results do not always indicate disease. The human body is very complex, and different results in different people can have different meanings. Therefore, interpretation and/or evaluation by your physician is essential.

Sample Forms for Ordering Laboratory Tests, Radiology Tests and Consults, Medical Supplies

■ REQUEST FOR RADIOLOGICAL EXAM ■

OPEN MRI
RADIOLOGY IMAGING SERVICES

2121 SALTWATER AVENUE, SUITE 100
MIAMI, FL 61312
(213) 475-6121 tel ▫ (213) 475-6000 fax

PATIENT NAME _____ AGE _____

APPOINTMENT DATE _____ Time _____

DIAGNOSIS _____

SPECIAL TECHNIQUE DESIRED _____

DOES PATIENT HAVE A HEART PACEMAKER OR INTRACRANIAL CLIPS?   ❑ YES   ❑ NO

MRI EXAMINATIONS	X-rays	

MRI EXAMINATIONS	Head	Spine
_____ MRA Extracranial	___ Skull-70260	___ Cervical-72050
_____ MRA Brain	___ Facial Bones-70150	___ w/Flex-Exten-72052
_____ Routine Brain	___ Nasal Bones-70160	___ Thoracic - 72070
_____ Post Fossa	___ Paranasal Sinuses-70220	___ Lumbosacral-72110
_____ Orbits	___ Mastoids-70130	___ Sacrum&Coccyx-72220
_____ Sella Turcica-Pituitary	___ Mandible-70110	___ Sacroiliac Joints-72202
_____ Neck	___ TMJs-70330	___ Pelvis-72170
_____ Cervical	___ Sella Turcica-70240	
_____ Thoracic	**Upper Extremities**	**Chest**
_____ Lumbosacral	R/L	___ PA/Lateral-71020
_____ Knee	___ Shoulder-73030	___ Ribs-71100/71110
_____ Hips	___ Clavicle-73000	___ Sternum-71120
_____ Shoulder	___ A.C. Joints-73050	___ Sterno clavicular-71130
_____ Ankle	___ Humerus-73060	
_____ Abdomen	___ Elbow-73080	**Abdomen**
_____ Pelvis	___ Forearm-73090	___ Flat-74000
_____ Chest	___ Wrist-73110	___ Upright-74000
_____ Other _____	___ Hand-73130	
_____	___ Finger-73140	
_____	**Lower Extremities**	
	R/L	R/L
	___ Hip-73510	___ Ankle-73610
	___ Femur-73550	___ Foot-73630
	___ Knee-73562	___ Toe-73660
	___ Leg-73590	

REFERRING
PHYSICIAN _____ DATE _____

TELEPHONE _____   STAT RESULT ❑ Yes ❑ No

On the Day of your MRI Scan . . . .

1. Follow your normal routine and take any medicine you regularly take. Do not wear makeup because some products may contain metallic particles.

2. Please arrive at OPEN MRI thirty (30) minutes before your appointment. Allow about 45 minutes for the procedure.

3. An OPEN MRI staff member will explain the procedure to you when you arrive.

The MRI procedure is performed in a room that holds a large magnet with a padded examination table. You will lie flat on the table that slides into the center of the magnet. While the imager is large and imposing, the procedure is quite simple and safe. When the machine is in operation, you will hear intermittent humming and thumping sounds. This is the normal sound of the equipment starting and stopping and other mechanical sounds.

The typical procedure takes an hour or less; however, the time required depends upon the part of the body being imaged. It is most important that you remain relaxed and still during the scan. You may resume your normal activities after the MRI is finished.

Pathology Laboratories

PLEASE PRINT WITH BLUE OR BLACK INK

Clinical Acsn Label

Patient Name - Last | First | M.I.

Patient I.D. | Room # | Phone/Add'l ID

Date of Birth — M M - D D - Y Y Y Y | Sex | Date M M D D Y Y | Time Collected H H : M M | ☒ AM ☒ PM

Requesting Physician | Fasting Y N | Urine Volume | ☒ STAT ☒ CALL ☒ Same Day

BILL ☒ MEDICARE ☒ CLIENT
TO: ☒ MEDICAID ☒ PATIENT
☒ PPO / POS ☒ HMO

LAB ___ ST ___ B ___ U ___ OP ___ GR
USE ___ L ___ SE ___ GP ___ SW ___ PR
ONLY ___ GY ___ F ___ HC ___ AF ___ OT

☐ 920 Venipuncture ☐ 925 Newborn Collection PSC ID
☐ 9999 Verbal Order ☐ 922 Ur Vol Meas
☐ 997 Verbal Diagnosis ☐ 940 Travel Phlebo ID
☐ 996 Standing Order ☐ Attachments

PLEASE COMPLETE INFORMATION BELOW

Responsible Party *REQUIRED* | Address *REQUIRED* | City, State, ZIP *REQUIRED* | Phone

Medicare/Medicaid Number *REQUIRED* | Insured SSN *REQUIRED* | Ordering Physician UPIN ■ R 5

Insurance Name | Member I.D. | Group

Insurance Address | City, State, ZIP | Phone

ADVANCE BENEFICIARY NOTICE (ABN): Medicare will only pay for services that it determines to be "reasonable and necessary" under Section 1862(a)(1) of the Medicare law. Screening procedures are excluded from the Medicare Program under Section 1862(a)(7). I have been notified that Medicare is likely to deny payment for laboratory tests specified below for the reason(s) stated.

Test Name

☐ **I will have the test(s) performed** and, if Medicare denies payment, I agree to be personally and fully responsible for payment.
☐ **I refuse to have the test(s) performed** since I am not willing to be responsible for payment.

✓ **Reason for probable Medicare payment denial:**
☐ this @ limited coverage test is not paid for with the diagnosis provided
☐ no diagnostic information was provided for this @ limited coverage test
☐ the test is considered "not medically necessary" under Medicare program standards
☐ the test is non-FDA approved or investigational
☐ the test is not paid at this frequency
☐ the test is for screening or is part of an annual physical exam

Date _____ Patient Signature _____

Physicians (or other individuals authorized by law to order tests) should only order tests that are medically necessary for the diagnosis or treatment of the patient. Physician or physician's staff shall provide ICD-9 codes, rather than narrative diagnoses, for each test or panel. **@ = Medicare Limited Coverage Tests.** See reverse page for additional Medicare limited coverage tests.

AMA Defined Panels (See Reverse for components) | ICD-9

9329	☒ General Health Panel Not covered by Medicare		ICD-9 Required
142	☒ Basic Metabolic Panel		
9179	☒ Comprehensive Metabolic Panel		
115	☒ Electrolyte Panel (NA, K, CL, CO₂)		
173	☒ Lipid Panel	@	ICD-9 Required
9175	☒ Liver (Hepatic) Function Panel		
514	☒ Obstetric Panel	@	ICD-9 Required
9324	☒ Kidney (Renal) Function Panel		
9325	☒ Acute Hepatitis Panel		
3270	☒ Drug Abuse Screen II *		

Tests | ICD-9

3800	☐ ABO & Rh Type		
3550	☒ ANA (Anti-Nuclear Abs) *		
2025	☒ Amylase		
2208	☒ BUN		
2209	☒ Calcium		
1000	☒ CBC with Differential with Platelets	@	ICD-9 Required
2645	☒ CEA	@	ICD-9 Required
3025	☒ Carbamazepine (Tegretol)		
2210	☒ Cholesterol, Total	@	ICD-9 Required
2075	☐ CK		
2214	☒ Creatinine		
3034	☒ Digoxin (Lanoxin)	@	ICD-9 Required
2675	☒ Estradiol		
2090	☒ Ferritin	@	ICD-9 Required
2695	☒ Folic Acid		
2700	☒ FSH		

2216	☒ Gamma GT		
2217	☒ Glucose	@	ICD-9 Required
2713	☒ HCG Quantitative	@	ICD-9 Required
2220	☒ HDL Cholesterol	@	ICD-9 Required
1041	☒ Hemogram w/o Differential with platelets	@	ICD-9 Required
1025	☒ Hemoglobin	@	ICD-9 Required
1030	☒ Hematocrit	@	ICD-9 Required
2708	☒ Hgb A1C (Glycohemoglobin)	@	ICD-9 Required
4565	☒ H. Pylori, IgG Ab, Qual.		
2725	☒ Hepatitis A Antibody *		
2739	☒ Hepatitis Bs Antigen		
2737	☒ Hepatitis Bs Antibody		
4675	☒ Hepatitis C Antibody		
3540	☒ HIV-1 Antibody	@	ICD-9 Required
2222	☒ Iron	@	ICD-9 Required
2118	☒ Iron + IBC	@	ICD-9 Required
2128	☒ Lithium		
2224	☒ LDH		
2776	☒ Luteinizing Hormone (LH)		
2130	☒ Magnesium	@	ICD-9 Required
3510	☒ Mono Screen		
3064	☒ Phenytoin (Dilantin)		
2228	☒ Potassium		
2714	☒ Pregnancy Test Serum Qual	@	ICD-9 Required
2800	☒ Prolactin		
2805	☒ Protein Electrophoresis		
2606	☒ PSA (Prostate Specific Antigen)	@	ICD-9 Required
2608	☒ PSA (Medicare Screen)	#	ABN Required

1425	☒ PT (Prothrombin Time)	@	ICD-9 Required
1430	☒ PTT (Partial Thrombo. Time)	@	ICD-9 Required
3505	☒ Rheumatoid Factor		
1055	☒ Sedimentation Rate (ESR)		
3500	☒ RPR*	@	ICD-9 Required
2218	☒ SGOT (AST)		
2219	☒ SGPT (ALT)		
2830	☒ Testosterone		
2817	☒ T3 Uptake	@	ICD-9 Required
2819	☒ T4, Total	@	ICD-9 Required
2823	☒ T4, Free	@	ICD-9 Required
2835	☒ TSH	@	ICD-9 Required
2233	☒ Uric Acid		
1501	☒ Urinalysis, Reflex Micro *		
3094	☒ Valproic Acid (Depakene)		
2840	☒ Vitamin B-12		

Microbiology: Source | ICD-9

4102	☒ Chlamydia DNA Probe		
4100	☒ GC DNA Probe		
6069	☒ Culture, Herpes		
6046	☒ Culture, Throat *		
6047	☒ Culture, Strep Screen		ABN Required
6043	☒ Culture, Stool *		
6049	☒ Culture, Urine *	@	ICD-9 Required
6052	☒ Culture, Vaginal *		
	☒ Culture ___ Source		
7015	☒ Occult Blood Screen (x3)	#	ABN Required
7000	☒ Ova & Parasites + Trichrome		

* If indicated, reflex testing will be performed with additional charge(s). # Medicare Frequency Limit. @ Medicare Limited Coverage Test.

3485

ADDITIONAL TEST (include ICD-9 Codes) / **SPECIAL INSTRUCTIONS:**

QUALI-CARE

OUTPATIENT LABORATORY REQUEST

Name:_____
    Last   First   M.I.
Address:_____

City:_____ State:_____ Zip:_____

Phone: (____)_____

D.O.B.:_____ SEX: ☐ M ☐ F SS #:_____

Religion:_____ Marital Status:_____

Physician:_____

Diagnosis/Code:_____

SPECIAL INSTRUCTIONS   ☐ STAT

☐ Call results to Physician at #:_____
☐ Preadmit Lab
☐ Surgery   Date:_____ Time:_____
                Location:_____
☐ _____

BILL TO: ☐ Patient   ☐ Physician's Account
            ☐ Insurance   ☐ Medicare/Medicaid

Insurance #:_____

PANELS/PROFILES	CHEMISTRY		COAGULATION
☐ 1-CBC, Master Chem	☐ Alk Phos	☐ Iron/TIBC	☐ APTT
☐ 2-CBC, Master Chem, T3,T4	☐ Amylase	☐ LDH	☐ Bleeding Time
☐ 3-CBC, Master Chem, T3, T4, TSH	☐ Bilirubin, Total & Direct	☐ Lipase	☐ Coagulation Profile
☐ Blood Smear Study	☐ BUN	☐ Lithium	☐ Fibrinogen
☐ Bone & Joint Panel	☐ C3	☐ Magnesium	☐ Prothrombin Time
☐ Chem 7	☐ C4	☐ Parathormone, C-Terminal	**BLOOD BANK**
☐ Chem 12	☐ Calcium	☐ Parathormone, Intact	☐ ABO & RH
☐ Chem 18	☐ Carbamazephine	☐ Parathormone, N-Terminal	☐ Antibody Screen, Indirect Coombs
☐ Chem 24	☐ CEA	☐ Phenobarbital	☐ Cold Agglutinins
☐ Electrolytes	☐ Cholesterol	☐ Phosphorus	☐ Rhogam (specify)
☐ Glucose Tolerance Test: _____ hrs.	☐ Cortisol ☐ AM ☐ PM	☐ Potassium	☐ Antenatal (_____ weeks)
☐ Healthy Heart Panel	☐ CPK	☐ Prostatic Acid Phosphatase	☐ Post-delivery
☐ Hepatitis Panel, Acute	☐ Creatinine	☐ Protein Electrophoresis	☐ Type and Screen for surgery within 72 hours
☐ Hepatitis Panel, Comprehensive (A,B,&C)	☐ Digoxin	☐ PSA	**SUBSTANCE ABUSE**
☐ Hypothyroid Panel	☐ Dilantin	☐ Salicylate	☐ 6 Panel Drug Screen
☐ Liver Function Panel	☐ Ferritin	☐ SGOT/AST	☐ 10 Panel Drug Screen
☐ Master Chem	☐ Folate	☐ SGPT/ALT	☐ Blood Ethanol
☐ Prenatal Profile, Comprehensive	☐ Glucose, 2 Hr Post Prandial	☐ Sjogren's Antibodies	☐ NIDA Drug Screen
☐ Prenatal Profile, Routine	☐ Glucose, Fasting	☐ T3 Uptake	☐ NIDA Look-alike
☐ Thyroid Profile	☐ Glucose, O'Sullivan	☐ T4-Thyroxine	**ADDITIONAL TESTS**
☐ Vitamin B12/Folate	☐ Glucose, Random	☐ Theophylline	
HEMATOLOGY	☐ Glycosylated Hemoglobin	☐ Triglycerides	☐ _____
☐ CBC w/Autodiff	☐ HDL Cholesterol	☐ TSH	
☐ Hematocrit	☐ Hepatitis B Surface AB	☐ Uric Acid	☐ _____
☐ Hemoglobin	☐ Hepatitis B Surface AG	☐ Valproic Acid	
☐ Reticulocytes	☐ HIV Screen	☐ Vitamin B12	
☐ Sed Rate	**MICROBIOLOGY**		☐ _____
☐ Hemoglobin Electrophoresis	Source:_____	☐ GC Smear	
URINE	☐ Acid Fast Smear Direct	☐ Gram Stain	
☐ Creatinine Clearance, 24 Hr.	☐ C. Difficile Toxin	☐ Occult Blood	☐ _____
☐ Urinalysis, Rout. (Microscopic if indicated)	☐ Chlamydia Antibody Test	☐ Ova & Parasites	
☐ Urinalysis with Microscopic	☐ Culture, Acid Fast**	☐ Pin Worm Slide	☐ _____
☐ Urine Pregnancy Test	☐ Culture, Anaerobic*	☐ Rotavirus	
SEROLOGY	☐ Culture, Blood*	☐ RSV	
☐ ASO	☐ Culture, Chlamydia	☐ Strep Screen Group A	☐ _____
☐ CRP	☐ Culture, Fungus	☐ Strep Screen Group B	
☐ FAN/ANA	☐ Culture, GC*	☐ Wet Prep/KOH	☐ _____
☐ HCG, Quant	☐ Culture, Routine*	☐ Wet Prep/Saline	
☐ Monospot	☐ Culture, Stool*	* Includes sensitivity with oral antibiotic panel if	
☐ RA Factor	☐ Culture, Throat*	pathogen found.	☐ _____
☐ RPR/VDRL	☐ Culture, Viral:	** Includes sensitivity if pathogen found.	
☐ Serum Pregnancy Test	Specify Type:_____	Please give antibiotic regimen:_____	
	☐ Fecal WBC		☐ _____
	☐ Fungus Smear		

WHITE COPY — Outpatient Lab   YELLOW COPY — Medical Record   PINK COPY — Physician/Patient

Send additional copy of report to:

☐ Call
☐ Mail

Physician's Address

Phone/Fax Number

City, State, Zip

1230.01

Patient's Name (Last)	(First)	Race	(MI)	Sex	Date of Birth MO DAY YR	Collection Time AM PM	Collection Date MO DAY YR

NPI / UPIN	Physician's ID #	Patient's SS #	Patient's ID #	Urine hrs/vol

Physician's Name (Last, First) | Physician's Signature

X_____

Medicare # (Include Prefix/Suffix)
☐ Primary
☐ Secondary

Medicaid # | State | Physician's Provider #

PATIENT

Patient's Address | Phone

City | State | ZIP

Name of Responsible Party (if different from patient)

Address of Responsible Party | APT #

City | State | ZIP

RESP. PARTY

Patient's Relationship to Responsible Party   ☐ 1 - Self   ☐ 2 - Spouse   ☐ 3 - Child   ☐ 4 - Other

INSURANCE

Insurance Company Name | Plan | Carrier Code

Subscriber/Member # | Location | Group #

Insurance Address | Physician's Provider #

City | State | ZIP

Employer's Name or Number | Insured SS# (If Not Patient)

Perform-ance Lab ☐	Carrier	Group #	Employee #	Mem

I hereby authorize the release of medical information related to the service described herein and authorize payment directed to LabCorp. I agree to assume responsibility for payment of charges for laboratory services that are not covered by my healthcare insurer.

X_____
Patient's Signature | Date

MEDICARE ADVANCE BENEFICIARY NOTICE (ABN)
I have read the ABN on the reverse. If Medicare denies payment, I agree to pay for the identified test(s).

X_____
Patient's Signature | Date

NOTE: WHEN ORDERING TESTS FOR WHICH MEDICARE OR MEDICAID REIMBURSEMENT WILL BE SOUGHT, PHYSICIANS SHOULD ONLY ORDER TESTS THAT ARE MEDICALLY NECESSARY FOR THE DIAGNOSIS OR TREATMENT OF THE PATIENT. BE SURE TO WRITE PATIENT'S NAME AND SOURCE OF SPECIMEN ON FROSTED END OF SLIDE IN PENCIL.

Diagnosis/Signs/Symptom in ICD-9 Format (Highest Specificity)

R E Q U I R E D

ICD-9 codes are the internationally accepted method of describing the clinical picture of the patient. All diagnoses should be provided by the ordering physician or his or her authorized designee. The following is a partial list of common diagnoses in ICD-9 format. Most third party payers require an ICD-9 code to indicate the medical necessity of the test(s) or profile(s) ordered. For a complete listing of all ICD-9 codes, please refer to a current ICD-9 manual.

V15.89	High Risk Cervical Screening	616.0	Cervicitis
V22.2	Pregnancy	616.10	Vaginitis
V76.2	Routine Cervical Pap Smear	617.0	Endometriosis, Uterus
180.0	Malignant Neoplasm, Cervix	622.1	Dysplasia, Cervix
		623.0	Dysplasia, Vagina
626.8	Abnormal Bleeding		
627.1	Post Menopausal Bleeding		
627.3	Atrophic Vaginitis		
795.0	Abnormal Cervical Pap Smear		

GYN-CYTOLOGY

† GYN Pap Smear   88164 ⓐ/P3000 %
009100 ☐ 1 Slide   009191 ☐ 2 Slides

† Vaginal Cuff Pap Smear   88164 ⓐ/P3000 %
009100 ☐ 1 Slide   009191 ☐ 2 Slides

† Pap Smear & Maturation Index 88155 ⓐ, 88164 ⓐ/P3000 %
009209 ☐ 1 Slide   190074 ☐ 2 Slides

† Liquid Based GYN Prep   88142 ⓐ/G0123 %
192005 ☐ Thin Layer Prep Pap Test

GYN Source - Check (✓)
☐ Cervical   ☐ Endocervical   ☐ Vaginal

Collection Technique - Check (✓)
☐ Brush / Spatula   ☐ Swab / Spatula
☐ Spatula Only   ☐ Brush Only
☐ Cervix Broom Only   ☐ Other

Required Information
Date LMP/Menopause

Previous Treatment - Check All That Apply (✓)
☐ None   ☐ Laser Vaporization
☐ Hysterectomy   ☐ Cryotherapy
☐ Conization   ☐ Radiation
☐ Colposcopy & Biopsy   ☐ Chemotherapy

DATES AND RESULTS _____

Check All That Apply (✓)
☐ Pregnant   ☐ Postpartum
☐ Lactating   ☐ IUD
☐ Oral Contraceptives   ☐ Postcoital Bleeding
☐ Postmenopausal Patient   ☐ DES Exposure
☐ Hormone Replacement Rx   ☐ Previous Abnormal Smear
☐ Postmenopausal Bleeding

NON-GYN-CYTOLOGY

009134 ☐ Breast Secretion   88160   ☐ Left
009092 ☐ Breast Aspiration   88172 88173   ☐ Right
009035 ☐ Bronchial Washing   88107
Lobe _____
009332 ☐ Bronchial Brushing   88104
Lobe _____
009076 ☐ Sputum   88108
009043 ☐ Pleural Fluid   88107
009050 ☐ Abdominal Fluid   88107
009068 ☐ Urine 88104   Voided ☐   Cath ☐
009001 ☐ Fine Needle Aspiration   88172, 88173
Source _____
009159 ☐ Misc. Fluid 88104   ☐ Synovial   ☐ CSF
Source _____
009126 ☐ Misc. Smear 88160   ☐ Herpes (Tzanck)
Source _____
009126 ☐ Labia / Vulva   88160
Pt History:

Admitting or Clinical Dx:

HISTOLOGY

Tissue / Source:
☐ Curettage   ☐ Biopsy   ☐ Excision   ☐ Re-excision

# of containers submitted _____   # received at lab _____

Preoperative Diagnosis:

Postoperative Diagnosis:

Clinical Impression:

Other Pertinent Clinical Data:
(Example: LMP __ / __ / __)

Accompanying Cytology   ☐ Yes   ☐ No

Additional Tests/Special Instructions:

Date, Spec#, & Dx of Previous Cytology/Histology: | Previously Submitted Material:

† Additional charge for physician-reviewed Pap Smears

LABORATORY REQUEST

PHYSICIAN:
_____

ADDRESS: _____

CITY: _____ STATE: _____ ZIP: _____

PHONE: (_____) _____

SPECIAL INSTRUCTIONS: ☐ STAT   ☐ FASTING

DATE COLLECTED: _____   TIME: _____ AM/PM

☐ CALL RESULTS TO PHYSICIAN AT: _____

☐

PHYSICIAN ICD-9 DIAGNOSIS REQUIREMENT NOTICE

When ordering tests, please be informed that the physician is required to make an independent medical necessity decision with regard to each test the laboratory will bill. Additionally, the physician understands he or she is required to (1) submit ICD9 diagnosis information (below), supported by the patient's medical record, as documentation of the medical necessity of the tests ordered and (2) explain and have the patient sign the Advance Beneficiary Notice Statement below if any of the tests marked by an & or any other tests for which Medicare is likely to deny payment are ordered.
NARRATIVE DESCRIPTION OF SYMPTOM/ DIAGNOSIS AND ICD9 CODE (MUST BE PROVIDED):

_____

_____

Physician Signature: _____

ADVANCE BENEFICIARY NOTICE (ABN) FOR MEDICARE PATIENTS: I have read the Advance Beneficiary Notice statement on the back of this request form and understand that, in my case, Medicare is likely to deny payment for services identified by an "&" below. If Medicare denies payment, I agree to be personally and fully responsible for payment.

X _____ Date: _____
PATIENT, PARENT OR GUARANTOR

PLEASE PRINT

PATIENT NAME: _____
    LAST   FIRST   MI

ADDRESS: _____

CITY: _____ STATE: _____ ZIP: _____

PATIENT PHONE: (_____) _____

DATE OF BIRTH: ____/____/____   SEX: ☐ M ☐ F

PATIENT SS #: _____ --- _____ --- _____

BILL TO: ☐ PATIENT   ☐ INSURANCE   ☐ PHYSICIAN / CLIENT
PLEASE PRINT   (COMPLETE BELOW)

	PRIMARY INSURANCE	SECONDARY INSURANCE
	☐ MEDICARE ☐ MEDICAID	☐ MEDICARE ☐ MEDICAID
INSURANCE CO:		
INSURANCE #:		
GROUP #:		
EMPLOYER:		
GUARANTOR:	Last First MI	Last First MI
RELATIONSHIP:		
INSURED SS#		

CONSENT STATEMENT: I hereby authorize to bill my insurance company and receive money for laboratory services provided and to release any of my medical records requested by the insurance company, and I agree to pay for any copayments, deductibles or non-covered services.

X _____ Date: _____
PATIENT, PARENT OR GUARANTOR

PANELS	AUTO CHEMISTRIES	INDIVIDUAL TESTS	INDIVIDUAL TESTS	MICROBIOLOGY
☐ **BASIC METABOLIC &** (80048) - Na, K, Cl, CO2, Glu, BUN, Creat, Ca	☐ ALBUMIN &	☐ ABO GROUP & Rh TYPE	☐ PREGNANCY, SERUM &	SOURCE: _____
☐ **COMPREHENSIVE METABOLIC &** (80053) - Na, K, Cl, Glu, BUN, Creat, Ca, TP, Alb, T Bili, AP, ALT (SGPT), AST (SGOT), CO2	☐ ALK PHOS &	☐ AMMONIA	☐ PREGNANCY, URINE &	COLLECTION TIME: _____
	☐ ALT (SGPT) &	☐ AMYLASE	☐ PROSTATE SPECIFIC AG (PSA) &	☐ CHLAMYDIA / GC, PROBE
	☐ AST (SGOT) &	☐ ANA	☐ PT (PROTHROMBIN TIME) &	☐ C. DIFFICILE TOXIN
☐ **ELECTROLYTE &** (80051) - Na, K, Cl, CO2	☐ BILIRUBIN, TOTAL &	☐ BLEEDING TIME	☐ PTT (PART.THROMBOPL. TIME)	☐ CULTURE, ACID FAST W/ SMEAR**
☐ **ARTHRITIS &** (80072) - Uric, RA, ESR, Fluor Ab Scr	☐ BILIRUBIN, DIRECT &	☐ CBC W/ AUTODIFF &	☐ RA SCREEN	☐ CULTURE, ANAEROBIC*
☐ **HEPATIC FUNCTION &** (80076) - AP, ALT (SGPT), AST (SGOT), Tot & Dir Bili, T Prot, Alb	☐ BUN &	☐ CEA &	☐ RPR &	☐ CULTURE, BLOOD*
	☐ CALCIUM &	☐ DIRECT COOMBS	☐ RUBELLA IGG	☐ CULTURE, ROUTINE W/ SMEAR*
☐ **HEPATITIS , ACUTE** (80074) - HAAb, HBcAb, HBsAg, HCVAb	☐ CHLORIDE &	☐ FIBRINOGEN	☐ SEDIMENTATION RATE (ESR)	☐ CULTURE, SPUTUM**
☐ **LIPID PANEL &** (80061) - Chol Total, Trig, HDL, LDL Calc	☐ CHOLESTEROL TOT&	☐ FOLATE	☐ T3 UPTAKE &	☐ CULTURE, STOOL*
	☐ CO2 &	☐ GLU TOLERANCE ___ HRS &	☐ THYROXINE (T4) &	☐ CULTURE, THROAT*
☐ **OBSTETRICAL &** (80055) - ABO/Rh, Ind Coombs, CBC, RPR, HBsAg, Rubella IgG Ab	☐ CK &	☐ GLYCOSYLATED HGB &	☐ TSH &	☐ CULTURE, URINE** &
	☐ CREATININE &	☐ HDL CHOLESTEROL &	☐ TYPE & SCREEN (FOR SURGERY WITHIN 72 HOURS)	☐ CULTURE, VIRAL SPECIFY TYPE: _____
☐ **RENAL FUNCTION &** (80069) - Alb, Ca, CO2, Cl, Creat, Glu, Phos, K, Na, BUN	☐ GLUCOSE, FAST &	☐ HEMATOCRIT &	☐ URINALYSIS, MICRO & CHEM	☐ GRAM STAIN
	☐ GLUCOSE, RAND &	☐ HEMOGLOBIN &	☐ URINALYSIS, REFLEX (MICROSCOPIC IF INDICATED)	☐ OCCULT BLOOD*
	☐ GGT	☐ HEPATITIS B SURFACE AB	☐ VITAMIN B 12	☐ OVA & PARASITES
	☐ LDH &	☐ HEPATITIS B SURFACE AG		☐ RSV
	☐ PHOSPHORUS &	☐ HEPATITIS C ANTIBODY	**TIMED URINE COLLECTIONS**	☐ STREP SCREEN GROUP A
	☐ POTASSIUM &	☐ HIV SCREEN	VOLUME: _____ ML	☐ STREP SCREEN GROUP B
	☐ PROTEIN, TOT &	☐ LIPASE	DURATION: _____ HOURS	* INCLUDES ID & SENSITIVITY WITH ORAL ANTIBIOTIC PANEL IF PATHOGEN IS FOUND.
	☐ SODIUM &	☐ MAGNESIUM &	☐ CREATININE CLEARANCE	** INCLUDES ID & SENSITIVITY IF PATHOGEN IS FOUND. LIST ANTIBIOTIC REGIMEN.
	☐ TRIGLYCERIDE &	☐ MEASLES, MUMPS, RUBELLA IGG	☐ PROTEIN	
	☐ URIC ACID	☐ MEASLES, MUMPS, RUBELLA, VARICELLA	☐ _____	

ADDITIONAL TESTS:

& = Medicare Limited Coverage Test

PATIENT ID# (LAB USE ONLY)

WHITE COPY – BHS MEDICAL RECORDS   YELLOW COPY – LABORATORY   PINK COPY – PHYSICIAN/PATIENT

Patient Name: _____

Referring Physician: _____

Diagnosis/Clinical History: _____

Appt. Date: _____ Appt. Time: _____

REPORTING INSTRUCTIONS :
- ☐ Report Only to Office
- ☐ Films with Report to Office
- ☐ Patient to Hand Carry Films
- ☐ Call Report : _____
- ☐ Fax Preliminary Report : _____

Follow Up Doctor Appointment Date: _____ Time: _____

Previous Films & Location: _____

MRI

☐ Intra-articular Gadolin   **☐ Contrast Enhancement**

- ☐ Brain
- ☐ Brain with IAC's
- ☐ Brain Spectroscopy
- ☐ Alzheimers
- ☐ Tumor
- ☐ Functional Brain
- ☐ Post Fossa
- ☐ Pituitary
- ☐ IAC's
- ☐ Orbits

- ☐ Chest
- ☐ TMJ
- ☐ Neck (Soft Tissue)
- ☐ C-Spine
- ☐ T-Spine
- ☐ L-Spine
- ☐ Cardiac MRI
- ☐ Morphology
- ☐ Cine
- ☐ Pericardium

- ☐ Abdomen*
- ☐ Pelvis*
- ☐ Pelvis (soft tissue)*
- ☐ Liver
- ☐ Prostate
- ☐ MRCP

☐ LEFT   **☐ RIGHT**   **☐ BILATERAL**

- ☐ Breast-Tumor
- ☐ Breast-Implant
- ☐ Shoulder
- ☐ Elbow

- ☐ Wrist
- ☐ Finger
- ☐ Hip only
- ☐ Hip w/ Limited Pelvis

- ☐ Knee
- ☐ Ankle
- ☐ Mid Foot
- ☐ Fore Foot

Other/Special Instructions _____

MRA

- ☐ Intracranial Arteries (Head)
- ☐ Extracranial Arteries (Neck)
- ☐ Dural Sinuses & Veins (Head)
- ☐ Portal Vein - Inf. Vena Cava
- ☐ CSF Flow Study

- ☐ Aorta - Abdominal
- ☐ Aorta - Thoracic
- ☐ Renal Arteries
- ☐ Femoral Arteries & Runoff

Other/Special Instructions _____

CT

CONTRAST: ☐ WO/W - IV*   **☐ IV***   **☐ NO ORAL***

- ☐ Brain
- ☐ Sinuses
- ☐ Sinuses Limited
- ☐ Temporal Bones/IAC's
- ☐ Orbits
- ☐ Facial Bones
- ☐ Neck Soft Tissue

- ☐ Chest
- ☐ Abdomen/Pelvis*
- ☐ Pelvis Only
- ☐ Upper Abd. Only*
- ☐ Liver
- ☐ Renal/Adrenals

- ☐ C-Spine
- ☐ T-Spine
- ☐ L-Spine
- ☐ 3-D Reformation
- ☐ Extremity _____

Other/Special Instructions _____

☐ Coronary Artery Calcium Scoring   **☐ Lung Cancer Screening**
☐ Whole Body Screening

NUCLEAR MEDICINE
(CLIA Certified)

- ☐ Bone Scan
- ☐ Total Body
- ☐ Limited
- ☐ 3 Phase
- ☐ SPECT
- ☐ Liver SPECT
- ☐ Liver/Spleen Scan
- ☐ RBC Liver Hemangioma
- ☐ Hepatobiliary (HIDA)*
- ☐ Cardiac MUGA Scan
- ☐ Meckels Scan*
- ☐ Gastric Emptying*
- ☐ Urea Breath Test (H-Pylori)
- ☐ Gallium Scan
- ☐ Indium Scan
- ☐ Lung Scan - Vent / Perfusion

- ☐ I-131 Whole Body Scan
- ☐ Thyroid Uptake
  - ☐ 6 hr.   ☐ 24 hr.
- ☐ Thyroid Scan
  - ☐ I-123   ☐ 99mc Tc
- ☐ Renal Scan
- ☐ Flow & Function
- ☐ Lasix Washout
- ☐ Captopril Challenge
- ☐ Residual Urine

THERAPY
- ☐ I-131 _____ mCi

NON-IMAGING PROCEDURES
- ☐ Dicopac (Schilling Test)
- ☐ Blood Volume

Other/Special Instructions _____

ULTRASOUND
(ACR Accredited)

- ☐ Abdomen*
- ☐ Abdominal Aorta*
- ☐ Gallbladder*
- ☐ Liver - Follow Up*
- ☐ Thyroid
- ☐ Kidney - Bilat.
- ☐ Kidney - ☐ LT ☐ RT
- ☐ Renal Transplant Eval.

- ☐ Pelvic*
  (with Trans-vaginal Ultrasound)
- ☐ Pelvic*
- ☐ Complete OB*
- ☐ Follow-up OB*
- ☐ Fetal Viability*
  (with Trans-vaginal Ultrasound)
- ☐ Hysterosonography*

- ☐ Testicular
- ☐ Prostate*
- ☐ Cyst Aspiration_

Other/Special Instructions _____

VASCULAR ULTRASOUND
(ICAVL Accredited)

   ☐ Arterial   **☐ Venous**

- ☐ Carotid
- ☐ Vertebral
- ☐ Doppler Aorta*
- ☐ Upper Extremity ☐ LT ☐ RT
- ☐ Lower Extremity ☐ LT ☐ RT
- ☐ Dialysis Graft Evaluation

- ☐ Abdominal Doppler*
- ☐ Hepatic*
- ☐ Renal*
- ☐ Mesenteric*
- ☐ Portal*

Other/Special Instructions _____

BONE DENSITY STUDY (DEXA)

- ☐ Osteoporosis Scan   Other/Special Instruction _____

✱ EXAMS THAT REQUIRE SPECIAL PREPARATION

MAMMOGRAPHY & BREAST DIAGNOSTICS

✱ Screening Mammogram - w/ return work-up and/or Ultrasound if indicated

- ☐ Diagnostic Mammogram
  (with Ultrasound if indicated)
- ☐ Implant Mammogram
  (with Ultrasound if indicated)
- ☐ Unilateral Mammogram ☐ LT ☐ RT
  (with Ultrasound if indicated)
- ☐ Breast Ultrasound ☐ LT ☐ RT
- ☐ Fine Needle Aspiration

- ☐ Cyst Aspiration
- ☐ Needle Localization
- ☐ Stereotactic Core Biopsy*
- ☐ Galactography
- ☐ Breast Scintigraphy (Miraluma®)
- ☐ Sentinel Node Localization

SPECIAL PROCEDURES

- ☐ Arthrogram*
- ☐ Discogram*
- ☐ Vertebroplasty
- ☐ Nerve Root Block*
- ☐ Facet Injection*
- ☐ Epidural Steroid (ESI)
- ☐ Lumbar Puncture

- ☐ Myelogram*
  - ☐ Cervical ☐ Thoracic ☐ Lumbar
- ☐ Joint Injection
- ☐ Venogram
- ☐ Hysterosalpingogram*
- ☐ Fallopian Tube Recanalization*

Other/Special Instructions _____

RADIOGRAPHY

HEAD
- ☐ Skull
- ☐ Facial Bones
- ☐ Mandible
- ☐ Sinuses
- ☐ Waters View

SPINE
- ☐ Cervical ☐ Thoracic ☐ Lumbar
- ☐ 5 Views   ☐ 3 Views
- ☐ AP & Lateral Only
- ☐ Flex & Extension
- ☐ Davis (7 Views)
- ☐ Scoliosis Study
- ☐ Sacrum/Coccyx
- ☐ Metastatic Survey

Other/Special Instructions _____

CHEST
- ☐ PA & Lateral
- ☐ Ribs ☐ LT ☐ RT
- ☐ Sternum

ABDOMEN
- ☐ Flat/Upright
- ☐ KUB

PELVIS
- ☐ AP

FLUOROSCOPY
- ☐ Esophogram
- ☐ Upper GI*
- ☐ Small Bowel
- ☐ Barium Enema*
  - ☐ W/ Air Contrast*
- ☐ IVP*
- ☐ VCUG
- ☐ Cystogram

☐ LEFT   **☐ RIGHT**   **☐ BILATERAL**

- ☐ Shoulder
- ☐ Humerus
- ☐ Forearm
- ☐ Elbow
- ☐ Hand
- ☐ Wrist
- ☐ Finger

- ☐ Femur
- ☐ Knee
- ☐ Tibia/Fibula
- ☐ Ankle
- ☐ Foot
- ☐ Toe
- ☐ Bone Age

- ☐ TMJ
- ☐ Clavicle
- ☐ Ribs
- ☐ Hip

Other/Special Instructions _____

RADIOLOGIC CONSULTATION REQUEST/REPORT
(Radiology/Nuclear Medicine/Ultrasound/Computed Tomography Examinations)

EXAMINATION(S) REQUESTED	AGE	SEX	SSN *(Sponsor)*		WARD/CLINIC	REGISTER NO.

FILM NO.

REQUESTED BY *(Print)*

PREGNANT   ☐ YES   ☐ NO

TELEPHONE/PAGE NO.

SIGNATURE OF REQUESTOR

DATE REQUESTED

SPECIFIC REASON(S) FOR REQUEST *(Complaints and findings)*

DATE OF EXAMINATION *(Month, day, year)*	DATE OF REPORT *(Month, day, year)*	DATE OF TRANSCRIPTION *(Month, day, year)*

RADIOLOGIC REPORT

PATIENT'S IDENTIFICATION *(For typed or written entries give: Name — last, first, middle, Medical Facility)*

LOCATION OF MEDICAL RECORDS

LOCATION OF RADIOLOGIC FACILITY

SIGNATURE

**RADIOLOGIC CONSULTATION
REQUEST/REPORT
1 — MEDICAL RECORD**

Building a Reference Library

Medical transcriptionists recognize the importance of maintaining a library of reference material. Keeping current is an ongoing and expensive effort; however, having current editions and up-to-date reference material is critical to the accuracy of medical transcription. Some considerations for building and maintaining a library of reference materials are as follows.

1. Build a basic library before branching out to the specialty areas, unless you happen to work in one of the specialty or subspecialty areas.

2. Have available both unabridged and collegiate editions of dictionaries, preferably with copyright dates within the past 5 years.

3. The word book(s) you choose should illustrate proper word division, i.e., hyphenation at the end of a line for both English and medical words.

4. Medical transcription is a mixture of technical writing and business writing—obtain reference books that will familiarize you with both areas.

5. Write to medical publishing companies and pharmaceutical companies and ask that your name be added to their mailing lists. Your local library will have addresses for companies that publish allied health reference material.

6. Read reviews of newly published editions and ask your peers, coworkers, and professional associates about them before you purchase additional reference books for your library. Some publishing companies offer a trial period on newly purchased volumes.

7. Before you purchase any dictionary or reference work, check for the most recent copyright date. Publishing company personnel can tell you if they plan to have a revision on the market soon; if possible, wait and purchase the new edition.

8. If you enroll in an anatomy, physiology, medical terminology, medical transcription, grammar review, proofreading or editing class, keep your textbooks because they are excellent reference books to add to your library.

9. Medical transcriptionists constantly edit and proofread; therefore, become familiar with the basics in these areas by enrolling in classes and obtaining and reading reference material. Learn the basic proofreading marks; they are printed in grammar reference books, style manuals, in some English dictionaries, and on page 190 in this appendix.

10. *Postal Addressing Standards,* the U.S. Postal Service publication 28, is available at no charge from the main branch of the post office. Business addressing standards are discussed in detail along with other important post office regulations.

Web Sites for Transcriptionists

American Association for Medical Transcription
http://www.aamt.org
Computer Systems Management
http://www.mtmonthly.com.
This site lists terms, drugs, instruments, and some specialties, such as AIDS terms and herbs used in alternative medicine.
Continuum Technologies
http://www.continuum-tech.com
Medical Transcription and Terminology Site
http://www.mtdesk.com
MedQuist: http://www.medquist.com
Medware: http://www.medware-inc.com
National Telecommuting Institute
http://www.nticentral.org
Spheris: http://www.spheris.com

General Interest Web Sites

American Arthritis Foundation: http://www.arthritis.org
American Autoimmune Related Diseases Association:
http://www.aarda.org
American Cancer Society: http://www.cancer.org
American Lung Association: http://www.lungusa.org
AWS: http://www.awsusa.com
Cancer News Site: http://www.cancernews.com
Drug Reference Site: http://www.eDrugInfo.com
Drug Reference Site: http://www.rxlist.com. Comprehensive listing of medications. You can even search by phonetic spelling or diagnosis to help you find the drug.
Flashcard Exchange www.flashcardexchange.com
Free online typing course: http://www.goodtyping.com
General Family Health: http://www.healthatoz.com
General Medical Information
http://www.medicinenet.com
General Medical Information: http://www.medscape.com
National Institute of Diabetes, Digestive, and Kidney Diseases: http://www.niddk.nih.gov
National Institute of Health—Bone Diseases
http://www.osteo.org
National Library of Medicine: http://www.nlm.nih.gov
National Stroke Association: http://www.stroke.org
Online Pharmacy: http://www.medexplorer.com
Search Engine: http://www.google.com
Ulcerative Colitis: http://www.living-better.com

A Healthcare Controlled Vocabulary

From Medical Abbreviations: 24,000 Conveniences at the Expense of Communications and Safety, *11th Edition, by Neil M. Davis (Huntingdon Valley, PA: Neil M. Davis Associates, 2003). Reprinted with permission.*

Presently there are no standards for physician's orders, consultations, written prescriptions, standing orders, computer order sets, nurse's medication administration records, pharmacy profiles, hospital formularies, etc. Because in the healthcare field everyone does their own thing, there are many variations. These variations in the way abbreviations are expressed are not always understood and at times are misinterpreted. They cause delays in initiating therapy, cause accidents, waste time for everyone in clarifying these documents, lengthen the time it takes to train those working in the healthcare field, lengthen hospital stays, and waste money.

A controlled vocabulary similar to what is used in the aviation industry is needed. Everyone in the aviation industry "follows the book," and uses a controlled vocabulary. All pilots and air traffic controllers say, "alpha", "bravo", "charley." They do not go off on their own and say "adam", "beef", "candy!" They say "one three," not thirteen, because thirteen sounds like thirty. Radio transmission in the aviation industry is not easy to decipher, yet because precision is critical everything possible is done to eliminate error. To prevent errors all radio transmissions are given only in English, every transmission is given in the same order, and must be immediately repeated by the receiver to make sure it was heard correctly. Written and oral communication in the medical professions are just as critical and are also not easy to decipher, so establishing a controlled vocabulary is also necessary in this industry.

Listed below are three organizations that have ongoing projects related to standardizing medical terminology:

Computer-Based Patient Record Institute, Inc.
1000 East Woodfield Rd. Suite 102
Schaumburg, IL 60173

The United States Pharmacopeial Convention, Inc.
12601 Twinbrook Parkway
Rockville, MD 20852

National Library of Medicine
Unified Medical Language System
8600 Rockville Pike
Bethesda, MD 20894

Listed below is the start of a Healthcare Controlled Vocabulary. The basis for this controlled vocabulary is established standard terminology and the result of 30 years of studying medication errors by this author.

It is anticipated that a Healthcare Controlled Vocabulary, with professional organizations' input and backing, will grow and some day evolve into an "official standard." Your suggestion and comments are vital to this growth and eventual recognition. It is always safest to avoid the use of abbreviations unless a standard has been established and is well publicized in your work environment.

Standard	What not to use or do	Comments
100 mg (100 space mg)	100mg (100 no space mg)	A United States Pharmacopeia standard way of expressing a strength is to leave a space between the number and its units. Leaving this space makes it easier to read the number as can be seen below. 1mg 1 mg 10mg 10 mg 100mg 100 mg
1 mg	1.0 mg	This is a USP standard. When a trailing zero is used, the decimal point is sometimes not seen thus causing a tenfold overdose. These overdoses have caused injury and death.
0.1 mL	.1 mL	When the decimal point is not seen, this is read as 1 mL, causing a tenfold overdose.

Standard	What not to use or do	Comments
once daily (Do not abbreviate)	The abbreviation OD The abbreviation QD	The classic meaning for OD is right eye. Liquids intended to be given once daily are mistakenly given in the right eye. When the Q is dotted too aggressively it looks like Q.I.D. and the medication is given four times daily. When a lower case q is used, the tail of the q has come up between the q and the d to make it look like qid. In the United Kingdom, Q.D. means four times daily.
unit (Do not abbreviate. Write "unit" using a lower-case u)	The abbreviation U	The handwritten U is mistaken for a zero when poorly written causing a tenfold overdose (i.e., 6 U regular insulin is read as 60). The poorly written U has also been read as a 4, 6 and cc. Write "unit," leaving a space between the number and the word unit.
mg (Lower case mg with no period)	mg., Mg., Mg, MG, mgm, mgs	The USP standard expression is the mg
mL (Lower case m with a capital L, no period)	mL., ml, ml., mls, mLs, cc	The USP standard expression is the mL
Use generic names or trademarks	Do not abbreviate drug names or combinations of drugs, such as CPZ, PBZ, NTG, MS, 5FC, MTX, 6MP, MOPP, ASA, HCTZ, etc. Do not use shortened names or chemical names	Abbreviated drug names and acronyms are not always known to the reader, at times they have more than one possible meaning, or are thought to be another drug. When the chemical name "6 mercaptopurine" has been used, six doses of mercaptopurine have been mistakenly administered. The generic name, mercaptopurine, should be used. When an unofficial shortened version of the name norfloxacin, norflox was used, Norflex was mistakenly given. An order for Aredia was read as Adriamycin, as some professionals abbreviated the name Adriamycin as "Adria" which looks like Aredia.
The metric system	The apothecary system (grains, drams, minims, ounces, etc.)	The apothecary system is so rarely used it is not recognized or understood. The symbol for minim (ɱ) is read as mL; the symbol for one dram (ʒт) is read as 3 tablespoons, and gr (grain) is read as gram.
Use properly placed commas for numbers above 999, as in 10,000, or 5,000,000	5000000	Many people have difficulty in reading large numbers such as 5000000. The use of commas helps the reader to read these numbers correctly.
600 mg When possible, do not use decimal expressions.	0.6 g	A USP standard. The elimination of decimals lessens the chance for error.
25 mcg	0.025 mg	Mistakes are made when reading numbers less than 1 with decimals.

CONTINUED		
Standard	**What not to use or do**	**Comments**
Do not use the term "bolus" in conjunction with the administration of potassium chloride injection. Use specific concentrations and the time in which the drug should be administered.		Some physicians will erroneously indicate that potassium chloride injection should be "bolused" or be given "IV push," vaguely meaning that it should not be dripped in slowly. Many deaths have been reported when prescribers have been taken literally and the potassium chloride was given by bolus or IV push. Orders should be specific such as, "20 mEq of potassium chloride in 50 mL of 5% dextrose to run over 30 minutes."
use "and"	Do not use a slash mark or the symbol "&"	A slash mark looks like a one. An order written "6 units regular insulin/20 units NPH insulin," was read as 120 units of NPH insulin. The symbol "&" has been read as a 4.
Orally transmitted medical orders should be read back as heard for verification	Do not assume that one has spoken or heard correctly.	During oral communications, speakers misspeak and/or transcribers mishear. To minimize these errors, the transmitter must speak clearly and slowly, the transcriber must repeat what was transcribed, and the transmitter must listen attentively when this is being done. This is less likely to occur when the prescription is complete.
When prescriptions are written or orally transmitted they must be complete. • dosage form must be specified • strength must be specified • directions must be specified • included in the directions must be the purpose or indication.	Incomplete orders	Prescribers on occasion think of one drug and mistakenly order another. Nurses and pharmacists on occasion misread prescriptions because of error, poor handwriting or poor oral communications, or look alike or sound alike drugs.[1] When the prescription is complete and the purpose or indication is included, these errors are less likely to occur. Listing the purpose or indication on the prescription label will assist in increasing patient compliance.
Written communications must be legible.	Illegible handwriting	Prescribers who cannot or will not write legibly must either print (if this would be legible), type, use a computer, or have an employee write for them and then immediately verify and sign the document.
Prescribe specific doses.	Do not prescribe 2 ampuls or 2 vials	There are often more than one size or concentration of drug available. Failing to be specific will lead to unintended doses being administered.
Establish a list of approved abbreviations with no abbreviation having more than one possible meaning within a context.	Everyone using their own abbreviations	To understand the scope of this problem examine the contents of this book for abbreviations that have many meanings and for obscure abbreviations that would not generally be recognized.
Use h or hr for hour	°	An order written as q 4° has been read as q 40 or the symbol ° has not been understood.

1. Davis NM, Cohen MR, Teplitsky BS. *Look-alike sound alike drug names: The problem and the solution.* Hosp Pharm 1992;27:95–110

Student Activities CD-ROM to Accompany
Hillcrest Medical Center: Beginning Medical Transcription Course, 6th Edition

Minimum System Requirements

Operating System: Microsoft Windows 98 SE, 2000, or XP

Processor: Pentium PC 500 MHz or higher (750Mhz recommended)

RAM: 64 MB (128 MB recommended)

Screen Resolution: 800 x 600 pixels

Color Depth: 16-bit color (thousands of colors)

Macromedia Flash Player V7.x. Macromedia Flash Player is free and can be downloaded from http://www.macromedia.com.

Installation Instructions

1. Insert disc into CD-ROM drive. The installation program should start up automatically. If it does not, go to step 2.

2. From My Computer, double-click the icon for the CD drive.

3. Double-click the setup.exe file to start the installation program.

Technical Support
Telephone: 1-800-477-3692, 8:30 AM–5:30 PM Eastern Time
Fax: 1-518-881-1247
E-mail: delmarhelp@thomson.com

StudyWare™ is a trademark used herein under license.

3.0 PROPRIETARY RIGHTS

3.1 The End User acknowledges that Thomson Delmar Learning owns all right, title and interest, including, but not limited to all copyright rights therein, in and to the Licensed Content, and that the End User shall not take any action inconsistent with such ownership. The Licensed Content is protected by U.S., Canadian and other applicable copyright laws and by international treaties, including the Berne Convention and the Universal Copyright Convention. Nothing contained in this Agreement shall be construed as granting the End User any ownership rights in or to the Licensed Content.

3.2 Thomson Delmar Learning reserves the right at any time to withdraw from the Licensed Content any item or part of an item for which it no longer retains the right to publish, or which it has reasonable grounds to believe infringes copyright or is defamatory, unlawful or otherwise objectionable.

4.0 PROTECTION AND SECURITY

4.1 The End User shall use its best efforts and take all reasonable steps to safeguard its copy of the Licensed Content to ensure that no unauthorized reproduction, publication, disclosure, modification or distribution of the Licensed Content, in whole or in part, is made. To the extent that the End User becomes aware of any such unauthorized use of the Licensed Content, the End User shall immediately notify Delmar Learning. Notification of such violations may be made by sending an Email to delmarhelp@thomson.com.

5.0 MISUSE OF THE LICENSED PRODUCT

5.1 In the event that the End User uses the Licensed Content in violation of this Agreement, Thomson Delmar Learning shall have the option of electing liquidated damages, which shall include all profits generated by the End User's use of the Licensed Content plus interest computed at the maximum rate permitted by law and all legal fees and other expenses incurred by Thomson Delmar Learning in enforcing its rights, plus penalties.

6.0 FEDERAL GOVERNMENT CLIENTS

6.1 Except as expressly authorized by Delmar Learning, Federal Government clients obtain only the rights specified in this Agreement and no other rights. The Government acknowledges that (i) all software and related documentation incorporated in the Licensed Content is existing commercial computer software within the meaning of FAR 27.405(b)(2); and (2) all other data delivered in whatever form, is limited rights data within the meaning of FAR 27.401. The restrictions in this section are acceptable as consistent with the Government's need for software and other data under this Agreement.

7.0 DISCLAIMER OF WARRANTIES AND LIABILITIES

7.1 Although Thomson Delmar Learning believes the Licensed Content to be reliable, Thomson Delmar Learning does not guarantee or warrant (i) any information or materials contained in or produced by the Licensed Content, (ii) the accuracy, completeness or reliability of the Licensed Content, or (iii) that the Licensed Content is free from errors or other material defects. THE LICENSED PRODUCT IS PROVIDED "AS IS," WITHOUT ANY WARRANTY OF ANY KIND AND THOMSON DELMAR LEARNING DISCLAIMS ANY AND ALL WARRANTIES, EXPRESSED OR IMPLIED, INCLUDING, WITHOUT LIMITATION, WARRANTIES OF MERCHANTABILITY OR FITNESS OR A PARTICULAR PURPOSE. IN NO EVENT SHALL THOMSON DELMAR LEARNING BE LIABLE FOR: INDIRECT, SPECIAL, PUNITIVE OR CONSEQUENTIAL DAMAGES INCLUDING FOR LOST PROFITS, LOST DATA, OR OTHERWISE. IN NO EVENT SHALL DELMAR LEARNING'S AGGREGATE LIABILITY HEREUNDER, WHETHER ARISING IN CONTRACT, TORT, STRICT LIABILITY OR OTHERWISE, EXCEED THE AMOUNT OF FEES PAID BY THE END USER HEREUNDER FOR THE LICENSE OF THE LICENSED CONTENT.

8.0 GENERAL

8.1 Entire Agreement. This Agreement shall constitute the entire Agreement between the Parties and supercedes all prior Agreements and understandings oral or written relating to the subject matter hereof.

8.2 <u>Enhancements/Modifications of Licensed Content</u>. From time to time, and in Delmar Learning's sole discretion, Thomson Thomson Delmar Learning may advise the End User of updates, upgrades, enhancements and/or improvements to the Licensed Content, and may permit the End User to access and use, subject to the terms and conditions of this Agreement, such modifications, upon payment of prices as may be established by Delmar Learning.

8.3 <u>No Export</u>. The End User shall use the Licensed Content solely in the United States and shall not transfer or export, directly or indirectly, the Licensed Content outside the United States.

8.4 <u>Severability</u>. If any provision of this Agreement is invalid, illegal, or unenforceable under any applicable statute or rule of law, the provision shall be deemed omitted to the extent that it is invalid, illegal, or unenforceable. In such a case, the remainder of the Agreement shall be construed in a manner as to give greatest effect to the original intention of the parties hereto.

8.5 <u>Waiver</u>. The waiver of any right or failure of either party to exercise in any respect any right provided in this Agreement in any instance shall not be deemed to be a waiver of such right in the future or a waiver of any other right under this Agreement.

8.6 <u>Choice of Law/Venue</u>. This Agreement shall be interpreted, construed, and governed by and in accordance with the laws of the State of New York, applicable to contracts executed and to be wholly preformed therein, without regard to its principles governing conflicts of law. Each party agrees that any proceeding arising out of or relating to this Agreement or the breach or threatened breach of this Agreement may be commenced and prosecuted in a court in the State and County of New York. Each party consents and submits to the non-exclusive personal jurisdiction of any court in the State and County of New York in respect of any such proceeding.

8.7 <u>Acknowledgment</u>. By opening this package and/or by accessing the Licensed Content on this Website, THE END USER ACKNOWLEDGES THAT IT HAS READ THIS AGREEMENT, UNDERSTANDS IT, AND AGREES TO BE BOUND BY ITS TERMS AND CONDITIONS. IF YOU DO NOT ACCEPT THESE TERMS AND CONDITIONS, YOU MUST NOT ACCESS THE LICENSED CONTENT AND RETURN THE LICENSED PRODUCT TO THOMSON DELMAR LEARNING (WITHIN 30 CALENDAR DAYS OF THE END USER'S PURCHASE) WITH PROOF OF PAYMENT ACCEPTABLE TO DELMAR LEARNING, FOR A CREDIT OR A REFUND. Should the End User have any questions/comments regarding this Agreement, please contact Thomson Delmar Learning at delmarhelp@thomson.com.